THE
IMMUNOTYPE
BREAKTHROUGH

THE IMMUNOTYPE BREAKTHROUGH

BALANCE YOUR IMMUNE SYSTEM,
OPTIMISE HEALTH AND BUILD
LIFELONG RESISTANCE

HEATHER MODAY, MD

First published in United States of America in 2021 by Little, Brown and Company, a division of Hachette Book Group, Inc.
This edition published in Great Britain in 2021 by Orion Spring
an imprint of The Orion Publishing Group Ltd
Carmelite House, 50 Victoria Embankment
London EC4Y 0DZ

An Hachette UK Company

10 9 8 7 6 5 4 3 2 1

A CIP catalogue record for this book is available from the British Library.

ISBN (Trade Paperback) 978 1 3987 0602 6
ISBN (eBook) 978 1 3987 0603 3
ISBN (Audio) 978 1 3987 0604 0

Typeset by Born Group
Printed and bound in Great Britain by Clays Ltd, Elcograf S.p.A.

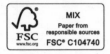

www.orionbooks.co.uk

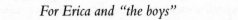

For Erica and "the boys"

Contents

THE
IMMUNOTYPE
BREAKTHROUGH

The Mystery of the Immune System, Our Body's Greatest Defense Mechanism

The year 2020 was a year we'll never forget, for so many reasons. For me, an immunologist and integrative and functional medicine expert, 2020 will always be the year when everyone started talking about the immune system. Terminology like "cytokines," "antigens," and "herd immunity" became commonplace lingo in socially distanced backyard gatherings.

Before COVID-19 hit, most of us probably didn't give our immune system a second thought, except maybe to figure that it helped us get over the common cold and back to work a little bit quicker; but all of a sudden, we started to look at it as a lifesaving mechanism in our body—a matter of life or death. And tragically, for many people throughout the course of the COVID-19 pandemic, the robustness of their immune system has been the determining factor between the two.

I wouldn't wish the year 2020 on anyone. But I can't help but feel that one positive that emerged was that we all started giving some respect and attention to the role our immune system plays in our lives. It is, after all, our body's greatest defense mechanism. It's what keeps you and me alive every day, no questions asked. But unfortunately, our immune system has long been taken for granted, ignored, and even abused.

Think about it: Every year we get screening tests for all kinds of things. We receive colonoscopies and mammograms to rule out cancer; we have cholesterol and blood pressure checks to analyze our cardiovascular health; some of us even get tested for nutrient deficiencies and have blood analyses for our liver and kidneys. But no one goes to their doctor and gets an immune system checkup. Just asking for that would likely generate a confused look and some head-scratching from your doctor.

Why is that? The immune system is clearly important—why don't we think about its general health and maintenance?

Part of the problem is that the human immune system is an enigma to much of the medical community, save for specialists and researchers. Quite honestly, I understand why. It's an incredibly complex system made up of innumerable cells, receptors, and chemical messengers that all seem to have intimidating names composed of perplexing numbers, letters, and symbols.

Not to mention, most doctors aren't taught that much about the immune system in medical school. Personally, I took a single immunology course in my second year of medical school and memorized enough facts to pass my exams. Had I not decided later to become an immunologist, I would have relegated most of that knowledge to the cobwebbed recesses of my brain, filed alongside the exact sequence of development of the fetal heart and the complex organic chemistry reactions I memorized (and then promptly forgot).

Another hurdle to understanding the immune system is the

massive amount of new research that has emerged in the past few decades. The field of immunology is evolving at a furious pace, constantly changing what we understand on a day-to-day basis. For a relatively young science—with origins in discoveries by the Russian scientist Élie Metchnikoff in 1883—the sheer volume of new information to keep up with is daunting for most doctors.

This truth was apparent in the way we scrambled as a society—rather, as a planet—to understand the SARS-CoV-2 virus and arm our immune systems to protect us from it. We all wondered what we should do to safeguard ourselves from infection with the virus. We donned masks, bought gallons of hand sanitizer, and socially distanced to the point of shutting down businesses, canceling holidays, and working from home for more than a year. We researched online whether certain supplements and dubious cures might protect us, and stayed glued to the news about the worldwide race for a vaccine. We heard about underlying conditions being a risk factor for bad outcomes and worried whether we were one of the vulnerable ones. We wanted to "boost" our immune systems but then learned that most people dying from COVID-19 suffered an *overactive* immune response called a cytokine storm. It's confusing, isn't it? So many questions and so few answers. It was enough to make us feel scared, overwhelmed, and as if our world was totally ill-equipped to handle an invisible microbe that spread like wildfire.

The fact is that supporting the immune system in the right way at the right time takes a little finesse. This is especially true when there's a novel threat, such as SARS-CoV-2. After all, there's no one reliable screening exam for our intricate and mysterious immune system. As you will discover in this book, our immune system is located in every nook and cranny of our body. It's a moving target and has no real boundaries or specified organs where it can be completely isolated and measured. You can't scan it with an X-ray, biopsy it, or determine its strength or weakness with a single test.

And even though we've been able to quickly develop effective vaccines for COVID-19, our immune systems will continue to face different challenges, such as new emerging viruses, throughout our entire lives! That's not where the threat to our immune system ends—not even close. Because even though we commonly associate the immune system with fighting off bacteria and viruses, the truth is that our immune system does way more than that. Its behavior—good or bad—influences or causes almost every disease known to humanity. The immune system is intricately involved in microbe-related illnesses like the common cold and flu, yes, but it is also a huge factor in heart disease, lung disease, diabetes, Alzheimer's, and cancer, which are the leading causes of death worldwide.

There is no other system in the body this elaborate and far-reaching. Essentially, the integrity of our immune system is the holy grail for the best quality of life. At the end of the day, its health determines whether we get sick and die of disease or enjoy hardy longevity.

When I started my career as an allergist and immunologist in private practice, I dutifully tried my best to tame the immune system. This was what I was trained to do. On a daily basis I treated eczema, hives, asthma, sinusitis, and occasionally a complicated immune disorder or deficiency. The treatments were standard—allergy shots, steroid injections, creams, allergy medications, asthma inhalers, and antibiotics. Most of the time, these methods helped for a while. But patients who'd left with a stack of prescriptions almost always came back in three to four months. As the years went on, I noticed that my patients were collecting new diagnoses, were getting sicker, and were ultimately taking too many medications, many of which were prescribed to help with side effects from other medications they were taking. Many complained of experiencing new food allergies as adults, autoimmune diseases, irritable bowel issues, rashes, chronic sinusitis, and joint pain. I began to get referrals from specialty doctors in gastroenterology, rheumatology, and dermatology, all stumped as to what to do next with their patients. (Allergists are often the doctors who get the complicated cases that no one else knows what to do with.) The problem was, despite years of conventional training in internal medicine, allergy, and immunology, I was baffled myself. But I had a hunch that all these new health issues were connected in some way.

So I just started asking questions. I inquired about my patients' nutrition, their stress levels, their daily routines, their emotions, their habits, and their sleep. Many of them didn't sleep well, had insomnia, or worked the night shift. Some had nutrient-poor fast-food diets and had been on multiple antibiotics and other prescription drugs in the past year. Others were depressed and stressed out or felt trapped in their relationships or unfulfilled in their jobs.

At this point, I was no expert in "integrative immunology," which I define as melding the hard laboratory science of immunology with the understanding of the factors that influence health, such as nutrition, stress, the mind–body relationship, environment factors, and spirituality, among others. I could clearly see that my patients' immune systems were suffering because of their lifestyles and behaviors. They were also getting the standard laundry list of diseases like high blood pressure, heart disease, and diabetes, which I knew had a strong immune component. I had no idea what to do to stop it besides writing more and more prescriptions. I needed a better toolkit.

I spent the next few years creating my own set of tools. I decided to complete an integrative medicine fellowship through the Dr. Weil Integrative Medicine program in Tucson to learn the benefits of various interventions like herbal medicine, nutrition, and repairing the mind-body connection. I attended functional medicine conferences, where I learned to focus not on naming diseases and covering up symptoms with medications but on searching for the root cause of disease using in-depth testing and evaluation, and then guiding patients through lifestyle changes to help heal themselves. I spent multiple weekends and vacations at these conferences all over the United States, digging into the science of what *really determines* whether we're sick or well, and I eventually got certified in functional medicine. I finally realized I couldn't integrate what I had learned into my current work situation, so I jumped ship from my job and embarked on my own, creating the Moday Center, a functional medicine practice in Philadelphia.

Since then I've worked with thousands of patients to reverse their health issues, including autoimmune disease symptoms, allergies, infections, and chronic diseases. Using tried-and-true protocols from my experience, I've helped them get off medications and feel better just by improving their environment, nutrition, microbiome health, sleep, and stress levels. I've helped patients reverse preexisting conditions and increase their resistance to viruses during the pandemic. I stocked my own unique toolkit, and I've put it to great use.

This book is that toolkit, distilled to a form that can be used by anyone, anywhere. In the following pages, you'll find a big chunk of the knowledge I've gained over the years, in a form that should be most useful to you. I've focused on what you *really need to know* about your intricate immune system and the practices that will help you become healthier and feel better. Because that's always the ultimate goal, right?

Over the past few years, I've read all the available advice for boosting immune health given by other health professionals—at conferences, on social media, and on medical websites—and realized it was all the same. As someone who has studied the immune system for decades, I can say with total certainty that this is not the right approach. Your immune system is not linear, and many things can go wrong to bring on disease; it's not as simple as just "boosting" immunity. You can develop chronic inflammation, autoimmune disease, and even issues like allergies, which are due to already-overzealous immune activity that would *not* benefit from an immune system "boost."

So what is the right approach? By helping hundreds of patients, I've learned that biochemical imbalances at the cellular level determine how the immune system goes awry and what symptoms we experience. During my years of research, I noticed several patterns emerging among my patients—and these became the blueprints for what I call the four Immunotypes: Smoldering, Misguided, Hyperactive, and Weak. In order to heal your out-of-balance immune system, you need to understand your specific Immunotype and then use specifically targeted lifestyle interventions and treatments to get yourself back on track.

That's why much of this book is centered around the four Immunotypes. We begin with the modern immune system crisis and an introduction to some of the underlying mechanisms that are fundamental to immune health. Then we'll be going back to class for a bit of Immunology 101. To understand your Immunotype, you have to speak a little of the language. Don't worry! It will be fun, and you can impress your friends at the next dinner party. After we've got the basics down, it's all about the four Immunotypes. I designed a self-assessment quiz to help you identify your unique Immunotype or Immunotypes (you can be more than one!) and present real-life case studies that help explain what's going on in the body for each. I'll explain how factors like sleep, stress, gut health, exposure to toxins, and nutrition affect your immune health and lead to imbalances. With this information and the knowledge of your specific type, you'll be able to craft your own Immune Restoration Plan that fits not only your Immunotype but also your lifestyle and preferences. The Immune Restoration Plan is the part of the book where we leave the classroom behind, roll up our sleeves, take action, and start restoring immune harmony.

If you follow the Immune Restoration Plan, you will squelch unwanted inflammation and redirect your immune efforts away from your own cells and harmless allergens and toward legitimate foes. You will build up your immune fortitude against novel viruses and bacteria and become a powerful fighter of cancerous cells. The ultimate goal with this book is to feel good and have confidence in your body. Because when your immune system is balanced, you feel fantastic! You rarely get sick, and if you do, you heal quickly. You're free of pesky allergies and don't suffer from autoimmune issues. You aren't battling diabetes, obesity, or heart disease, or dealing with other chronic inflammation. Your immune system has resilience, and as a result, so do you.

So, whether you want to fend off chronic disease, get your autoimmune symptoms under better control, or free yourself from annoying seasonal allergies or constant colds or sinus infections, this book will provide you with your own toolkit to do just that.

Time and time again, I have seen the human body's miraculous ability to heal. And I know that you can experience this, too. Your immune system wants to protect you, but as you'll learn in this book, it can do its job only with your support.

What do you say? Are you ready to become your own immune system expert? Turn the page to get started.

Part I

THE AGE OF IMMUNE IMBALANCE

CHAPTER 1

The Immune Dysfunction Crisis

During the summer of 1906 in the exclusive enclave of Oyster Bay, New York, a banker and his family were enjoying their summer vacation on the shore, swimming, tanning, and having picnics. Midway through the summer, though, a terrible sickness broke out. Fever and diarrhea disrupted their idyllic respite, and six of the eleven occupants of the house fell ill with infectious gastroenteritis. The culprit was later revealed to be *Salmonella typhi,* the bacterium responsible for typhoid fever.

Although they usually only affected those living in cities with contaminated water and poor sanitation, typhoid outbreaks started popping up in similarly affluent households over the next few years. After much investigation, the illnesses were traced back to a single person—a hired cook named Mary Mallon, infamously referred to as Typhoid Mary.[1] It turned out that Mary was an asymptomatic carrier of the disease, and she effectively spread this sometimes lethal infection to her unsuspecting clientele in house after house, year after year.

This was the age in America before antibiotics, vaccines, mass sanitation, public water treatment, hygienic food handling, and proper sewage disposal. And the truth is, this age wasn't that long ago! At the turn of the twentieth century, the most common causes of death were infectious diseases like pneumonia and influenza, tuberculosis, and infectious gastroenteritis. In fact, in 1900, the average life expectancy in the United States was only forty-seven years.[2] Let that sink in. Just a little over a hundred years ago, we did not have safe or reliable vaccines, Alexander Fleming had yet to discover penicillin, and we didn't have a solid understanding of how we actually got infections. In fact, surgeons didn't routinely start washing their hands before surgery until the late 1800s, and wearing masks and gloves during medical procedures wasn't commonplace until the turn of the twentieth century.

As a result, many infections we prevent with vaccines or treat with a simple round of antibiotics today ended in death, especially in children. Today we take for granted all the amazing medical advances at our fingertips, but in the past, a strong immune system was the only protection in the battle against a potentially fatal infection.

THE INFECTIOUS-TO-CHRONIC DISEASE PIVOT

In the past hundred years, we've done a complete 180-degree pivot. Can you name a friend or family member who has died of a stomach bug, syphilis, or tuberculosis? That's not to say that infectious diseases are a thing of the past—far from it, as we've seen with the AIDS epidemic of the 1980s, the recent global COVID-19 pandemic, and the rise of antibiotic-resistant "superbugs"—but modern society, our food industry, medical technology, and human behavior have radically altered why we get sick and how we die.

With the exception of the specter of novel viruses rising in our future, the threat of infectious disease just isn't what it used to be.

This is thanks, in large part, to vaccines. As recently as 1960, there was no nationwide vaccine initiative, and children received just five vaccines for diphtheria, tetanus, pertussis, poliomyelitis, and smallpox. Since then there's been an explosion in vaccine development, with sixteen vaccines routinely given to all children, spread out via fifty-six injections over eighteen years. Regardless of your stance on vaccines, these innovations certainly have drastically decreased childhood mortality from infections, which is definitely something to celebrate, but now it seems we're facing an entirely different crisis—a sharp rise in chronic disease. We're living far longer than we used to, but we're also chronically sicker than we've ever been. In fact, we've developed an immune dysfunction crisis.

This is our reality: Kids are being diagnosed with asthma, food allergies, diabetes, hypertension, autism, and ADHD at rates unlike anything we've ever seen before. In the US and worldwide, diseases like heart disease, lung disease, diabetes, Alzheimer's, and cancer top the list of what kills us.

The statistics don't lie. Currently:

- Cardiovascular disease—including coronary artery disease, congestive heart failure, stroke, arrhythmia, high blood pressure, and peripheral artery disease—affects 48 percent of the US population and is the leading cause of death worldwide.[3]
- About 34.5 million Americans have been diagnosed with type 2 diabetes, a disease that can lead to blindness, kidney dialysis, stroke, heart disease, and limb amputation.[4] Even more staggering, add on people with prediabetes or undiagnosed diabetes and you're at 100 million Americans.[5] That's

one in three people walking around with a blood sugar problem.

- Alzheimer's disease affects close to 6 million people in the United States and is expected to rise to more than 15 million by 2050.[6] That means there will be more Alzheimer's patients than people living in New York City, Chicago, and Los Angeles combined.

- The prevalence of obesity among US adults was 42.4 percent in 2018, which is about double what it was when I was a college freshman thirty years ago. Obesity on its own raises your risk for heart disease, diabetes, dementia, and arthritis.[7]

- Anxiety disorders and depression are rising dramatically too. Even before the COVID-19 pandemic, a whopping 18.5 percent of adults suffered from anxiety or depression. That number is now almost certainly higher.[8]

- According to the National Institutes of Health, autoimmune disease affects 23.5 million Americans (that's more than 7 percent of the population), and the American Autoimmune Related Diseases Association (AARDA) estimates that the number is actually closer to 50 million Americans.[9]

- The most recent Centers for Disease Control and Prevention (CDC) statistics cite 47 percent of Americans having at least one type of chronic disease, which costs the country $3.7 trillion a year.[10]

I feel like we have become numb to the information above. There's little shock value to it anymore because it's so normalized. But believe me, it's far from normal.

Chronic disease is tricky because unlike an infectious disease that can leave us bedridden for days with a fever, chills, or diarrhea, chronic disease is sometimes harder to spot. Take a second to think about the people you know: How many of them suffer from a chronic condition like psoriasis, high blood pressure, irritable bowel syndrome, or endometriosis? You wouldn't necessarily even know unless they told you. I'm always surprised by how often I'll be chatting with a friend or family member and all of a sudden they mention that they have rheumatoid arthritis, asthma, or ulcerative colitis. Somehow I still naïvely think, "How is this the first time I'm learning this?"

The answer is simple: Sickness looks very different these days. You can't always detect chronic illness on the surface, and given the plethora of drugs we have, we can sometimes "control" disease. But that doesn't always mean we're feeling well or living well. In fact, the major effort in conquering chronic disease hasn't been in eliminating its root causes but instead in sinking billions of dollars into developing ever-more-potent drugs.

The statistics on prescription drugs don't lie, either:

- 45.8 percent of the US population has used prescription drugs in the past thirty days, 24 percent of Americans have used three or more, and 12.6 percent of Americans have used five or more.[11]
- 18.0 percent of children zero to eleven years old have taken a prescription drug in the last month.
- 73.9 percent of doctor visits involve prescribing drugs, according to the CDC.[12]
- About 13.2 percent of Americans aged eighteen and over have taken an antidepressant medication in the past thirty days.[13]
- The prevalence of the use of NSAIDs (non-steroidal anti-inflammatory drugs—over-the-counter pain relievers) in

patients over sixty-five years old is as high as 96 percent in some settings.[14]

- More than 16 million opioid prescriptions were written in 2018, and roughly 21 to 29 percent of the patients prescribed opioids end up misusing them, with 12 percent developing an addiction.[15]

- Overall, the use of statin drugs for cholesterol among US adults forty years of age and older in the general population increased 79.8 percent, from 21.8 million individuals in 2002–2003 to 39.2 million individuals (27.8 percent) in 2012–2013 (that's 221 million prescriptions).[16]

- More than 15 million Americans have prescriptions for PPIs (proton pump inhibitors — common drugs used to lower stomach acid) to control heartburn (even more surprising, research has shown that as many as 10.5 million people take PPIs even when they don't need them).[17] [18]

- According to the CDC, 16 million adults use allergy medications, and more Americans are buying allergy medications every year.[19]

Prescription and over-the-counter drugs are not inherently bad — in fact, they can be extremely helpful — but the truth is, they've only been marginally successful in solving the problem of chronic disease. While many of these medications are lifesaving and can reduce symptoms, they can also have deleterious side effects and addictive qualities, and don't usually address the underlying cause of the health issue, which means you inevitably end up back at the doctor needing a higher dose or another drug. Many people are living in states of persistent illness, pain, disability, and substandard quality of life.

You might be wondering why I'm talking about all these different diseases and medications. They can't all be connected to the immune system, can they? Actually, they can and they are. In fact, I would go as far as to say that most chronic illnesses are a cry for help from our immune systems. A cry for help that takes the form of chronic systemic inflammation.

THE DOUBLE-EDGED SWORD OF INFLAMMATION

Recently I had a client show up in my office and say, "I don't know what's wrong. I just feel so off." Although she didn't have a specific diagnosis, she knew something wasn't right. As I mentioned, diseases ranging from depression to heart disease to Alzheimer's to inflammatory bowel disease all are driven by an issue with the immune system—and that issue is almost always inflammation. You're likely going to get sick of hearing this word, because you'll hear it again and again throughout the course of this book, but that's because it's the linchpin of the immune system. In fact, whenever we're injured or infected, the first thing our immune system does is trigger the inflammatory cascade as a counterattack.

Inflammation tends to get a bad rap, especially in the wellness world, but it's somewhat misunderstood. Because inflammation isn't all bad! In fact, if we didn't have inflammation, we'd die from mild infections like the common cold or flu or even from minor wounds because our body wouldn't be able to protect and repair itself.

Here's what I mean: When your body gets injured or infected, the immune system triggers an inflammatory response to send an army of immune cells and other chemical messengers to the area to protect and heal it (we'll learn about these cells and messengers more in Chapter 2). Inflammation is what causes swelling, redness, and heat when we injure ourselves, and it's what causes the overproduction of mucus when we get a cold. All of these things annoy us and make us feel bad, but they're actually there to heal and help us banish infectious germs from our bodies. A swollen, painful ankle keeps us from walking around reinjuring it again and again; the mucus we produce and cough up when we have a cold is there to capture and expel the germ that got us sick.

In a perfect world, the inflammation caused by an injury or illness would be short-lived, would be appropriate for the size and severity of the threat we were facing, and would succeed in initiating protection and healing before it died out and our body went back to its normal state. Unfortunately, it doesn't always go this way. Sometimes, our inflammatory response gets triggered too much and the inflammation produced can become more serious than the original illness or injury—for instance, in the case of cytokine storms from COVID-19; other times, inflammation does not subside properly after the threat has passed. When this happens, it's bad news for the body and can create—yes, you guessed it!—a chronic inflammatory state that leads to chronic disease. Today, an overwhelming number of diseases stem from simmering low-level inflammation, and we have boatloads of it.

For example:

- In atherosclerosis, the plaque that builds up and eventually calcifies our heart and blood vessels is a result of our immune systems' attempts to create inflammation to repair damage to the blood vessels themselves. The plaque grows from insults like smoking, infections, high blood pressure, toxic chemicals, and damaged cholesterol.
- Depression has been connected to higher levels of inflammation affecting neurotransmitter function in the brain.[20]

- In diabetes, inflammation spins out of control when excess blood sugar sticks to blood cells and blood vessels, damaging organs that we frantically try to repair.
- As for Alzheimer's disease, your risk of developing the condition increases with environmental toxins, concussions, high blood sugar, and lack of sleep. These are all drivers of—you guessed it again!—inflammation, which results in an overrepaired and damaged brain.
- Asthma is inflammation of the airways, eczema is inflammation of the skin cells, arthritis is inflammation of the joints, and Crohn's disease is inflammation of the digestive tract—the list could go on and on.

Clearly, an inflammatory response that's spun out of control is at the root of many common illnesses. This is especially true for a group of conditions called autoimmune diseases.

IMMUNE "TOLERANCE" AND AUTOIMMUNE DISEASE

As we learned earlier, autoimmune diseases are a family of chronic, debilitating, and sometimes life-threatening disorders. And what they all have in common is an immune system that has gone haywire. This creates a ton of chronic inflammation, but it also leads to a breakdown of the intelligence of the immune system so that it starts attacking the body's own tissues as if they were dangerous outside invaders. In immunology-speak, we call this phenomenon the loss of "tolerance," which is a key concept in immunology. Tolerance is basically the ability of your immune cells to recognize your own tissue and never attack it. When you lose immune tolerance, your immune cells start attacking your tissues. A loss of tolerance is one of the factors in developing autoimmune disease (autoimmunity) and what I have named a Misguided Immunotype, which you'll learn more about later.

Autoimmunity can occur anywhere, but the most common locations are the blood vessels, connective tissues, endocrine glands such as the thyroid or pancreas, joints, muscles, red blood cells, and skin. Some of the most common autoimmune diseases are:

- Addison's disease
- Celiac disease — sprue (gluten-sensitive enteropathy)
- Dermatomyositis
- Graves' disease
- Hashimoto's thyroiditis
- Multiple sclerosis
- Myasthenia gravis
- Pernicious anemia
- Reactive arthritis
- Rheumatoid arthritis
- Sjögren's syndrome
- Systemic lupus erythematosus
- Type 1 diabetes

You probably know someone with one of the conditions above, and you may never have thought about the fact that it's an autoimmune condition. Take rheumatoid arthritis (RA), for example. You may think of this condition as just pain and stiffness in the joints, but it's much more than that. RA results when immune cells mistakenly attack the body's own healthy joints, causing pain, deformity, and swelling. Inflammation is both an underlying cause and a side effect of autoimmunity, and it creates a vicious cycle of inflammation–autoimmunity–more inflammation in the body that can quickly take over your life. I'll talk more about autoimmunity later on when we talk about the Misguided Immunotype, but for now just remember that quelling chronic inflammation will be a big part of the Immune Restoration Plan. Why? Because chronic inflammation can be triggered by many aspects of our internal and external environment, especially those aspects that are too small for us to even see. In the next section, we'll be going microscopic to talk about just how much microbes still rule our life and health, even though the typhoid fever days are behind us.

THE "OLD FRIENDS" HYPOTHESIS EXPLAINED

Remember when I said we've done a 180-degree pivot and traded infectious disease for a chronic disease epidemic? Well, a lot of people think our obsession with "killer germs" has gone way too far and has led to this unbelievable rise in chronic disease. In 1989, an inconspicuous journal article written by epidemiologist D. P. Strachan made a major statement. The article linked hay fever and eczema in children to smaller family size and fewer childhood infections. Strachan's theory was essentially this: The fewer infections you had as a child, the more allergies you developed later on. This idea became wildly popular among both scientists and the news media and was quickly dubbed the "hygiene hypothesis."[21] Besides having a nice ring to it, the hygiene hypothesis was centered around the idea that our increasingly antiseptic environment—thanks to disinfectants, antibiotics, hand sanitizer, and investments in clean water, public sanitation, and personal hygiene practices—has put us at higher risk for allergic diseases and a "Hyperactive Immunotype," which is characterized by an over-the-top allergic response.

The hygiene hypothesis does have some truth to it—we've focused so much on preventing and treating infectious diseases caused by pathogenic microbes, we've gone a little too far and it's ended up backfiring. The hygiene hypothesis says that this lack of exposure paves the way for an immune system that is so used to an oversterilized environment, it ends up attacking everything it's exposed to, even if that thing is harmless, like pollen or dust. There's also evidence to support this hypothesis, like the fact that there has been a huge uptick in asthma and allergies over the past thirty years. And it's true that this surge has occurred almost exclusively in Westernized, wealthier, more technologically advanced countries that have also become increasingly "hygienic." But here's my take: The hygiene hypothesis isn't 100 percent accurate. Why? Because as we saw with the COVID-19 pandemic, we shouldn't be throwing out our soap and Lysol wipes anytime soon. It's just not that simple. A more valid and inclusive explanation of why we have all these allergies is the "Old Friends Hypothesis" put forward by physician and microbiologist Dr. Graham Rook.[22]

This spinoff hypothesis says that it's not the dangerous microbes that frame our developing immune system, but rather the "commensal" microorganisms—including beneficial bacteria, fungi, protozoa, and viruses—that have coexisted in our bodies for millennia. These beneficial microbes influence our health in more ways than we can possibly imagine. You've probably heard that there are bacteria in your digestive tract, which is often referred to as the "gut microbiome," but the truth is, we have "good bugs" colonizing our skin, mouth, sinuses, lungs, and other parts of the body as well. There are trillions of them; in fact, the number of bacterial genes in a human's microbiome is 200 times the number of actual human genes in the body.

So where do all these "old friends" come from? Before we're born, we exist in the sterile environment inside our mother, but as soon as we make our way out of the womb (whether through the birth canal or via cesarean section), we start picking up these friendly bugs and our microbiome starts developing. Pretty soon after that, we start getting beneficial microbes from breast milk and cuddling with our parents, and eventually from lying on the grass, having a dog or cat, playing in the dirt, and even having siblings (more people means more bacteria!). If you've ever wondered why doctors recommend vaginal deliveries and breastfeeding as much as they do, it's all about exposing the baby to these beneficial microbes right away to promote healthy microbiome development.

Healthy microbes help shape our immune system positively and encourage immune cells called regulatory T cells. We'll talk more about exactly what these cells do in the next chapter, but for now, just know that friendly microorganisms coach our regulatory T cells to be more "tolerant" of our environment, which helps us avoid allergies, autoimmunity, and chronic inflammation. Knowing this, you can see why many researchers and scientists are concerned that an overly sterile birth and childhood—devoid of time playing in the dirt and petting animals, and full of hand sanitizer and Lysoled surfaces—can sabotage the development of immune tolerance. On a positive note, as you'll learn in Chapter 7, we don't need to live in total filth as children, be sick all the time, or never wash our hands again in order to support these microbes. Instead, we can focus on protecting ourselves from dangerous germs through reasonable sanitation practices—especially in situations like the COVID-19 pandemic, where we've been faced with a novel virus to which we have no immunity—while also making sure we get plenty of exposure to "good bugs."

One of the biggest challenges to rebalancing your immune system—whether you have a Smoldering, Misguided, Hyperactive, or Weak Immunotype—is to establish a healthy relationship with the 38 trillion bacteria currently residing in your body. As humans, we need to start showing these microbes some respect and allow them to do their job; otherwise, our immune systems don't stand a chance! The good news is that later in this book there's an entire chapter on how to live more symbiotically with the microorganisms that inhabit our bodies.

THE AXIOM OF "BOOSTING"

As we just learned, taking an oversimplified approach to microbes — by simply trying to "kill all germs" — has backfired. Unfortunately, we often fall victim to the same thinking when it comes to optimizing the health of the immune system. If I had a dollar for every time I read an article, blog post, or product advertisement singing the praises of "boosting" your immune system, I'd be able to retire next year and move to a luxurious tropical island. Let me be clear: There are some situations where boosting your immune response might be beneficial, such as in the case of a Weak Immunotype, but you have to know what parts of the system you're boosting, how much, and in what way. Just focusing on increasing the activity of the immune system is not always a good thing. For example, if you have allergies or asthma, your symptoms stem from an immune system that's already hyperactive, and the last thing it needs is a "boost." Some of us have vigorous immune responses that end up attacking our own tissues, and we'd benefit from less immune activity, not more. The point I'm trying to make here is that there's no one-size-fits-all approach to boosting your immune system — that would be a grave insult to the spectacular intricacy of how this system functions in the human body. It would also ignore the distinctive characteristics of each person's imbalances. You have to have a sense of where you are in order to know where to go.

This need for more specificity and better-informed decisions is what has guided much of the content in this book. My goal is to help you find out where you fall on the spectrum of immune dysfunction, which is another way of saying identify your Immunotype. Only when you've identified your Immunotype will you have a better sense of whether you need to boost, calm, or redirect your immune response. And here's where it gets even more complicated: Your immune system doesn't always become imbalanced in just one way. When you take the Four Immunotypes Quiz later on in this book, you may find that you land on more than one Immunotype. Not only is that normal, it's common. Immune dysfunction has a domino effect, and once you get imbalanced in one area, you often unravel in another.

THE GOOD NEWS — NURTURE > NATURE

So far in this chapter, I've delivered a lot of scary statistics, harsh realities, and, let's be honest: bad news. We are no doubt in the middle of an immune dysfunction crisis that deserves our immediate attention.

But it's not all bad news. Why? Because as with most systems in the body, our immune system is in a state of constant flux. Billions of immune cells die, transform, and are born every second, and that means we have daily (even hourly!) opportunities to transform the integrity and resilience of our immune health. We do this by making changes in our lifestyles, diet, habits, and environment. Many of my patients look skeptical when I tell them this. I get it! If you're suffering from lifelong allergies, an autoimmune disease, or a chronic illness, it can feel like things are totally out of your control. And after reading this chapter up until this point, you may also feel like all the oversanitizing, overmedi- cating, and "boosting" our society has been doing means we have a lot to unlearn and a lot of ground to make up. But I assure you that even if you came into the world immunologically disadvan- taged, even if you're suffering from a disease that disrupts your life on a daily basis, even if you've been doing everything wrong for your immune system until right now, you have the capacity to reshape and revise your own immune behavior.

Why am I so sure? Because not only have I witnessed hun- dreds of patients balance their immune systems with diet and life- style changes, I've also seen study after study connect all types of immune health issues to factors that are very much under our control. If you've been living mostly in the conventional medi- cine world until now, this might be the first time you're hearing all of this, and if you're skeptical, I understand. Many doctors, even specialists, are still woefully uninformed on the impact of lifestyle interventions. Most doctors get fewer than twenty-five hours of nutrition training in four years of medical school, and fewer than 20 percent of medical schools have a single required course in nutrition.[23] As someone who went to medical school and found myself in practice unable to support my patients in this way, I know better than anyone.

One of the biggest issues with this is that it has relegated nutri- tion, exercise, and mind-body interventions to the "woo-woo" category of health care, reserved for so-called "alternative medi- cine" practitioners. We love to poke fun at yogis and green juice drinkers and crystal lovers, but I'm here to tell you that there's absolutely nothing "woo-woo," crazy, or unsubstantiated about true lifestyle medicine.

The research doesn't lie: One groundbreaking study showed

that just four healthy lifestyle factors—not smoking cigarettes, maintaining a healthy weight, exercising regularly, and following a healthy diet—together can reduce your risk of developing the most common and deadly chronic diseases by 80 percent. *Read that again—80 percent.*

Not to mention:

- Consuming ten portions per day of fruits and veggies could prevent about 7.8 million premature deaths worldwide each year.[24]
- Stress plays a part in 75 percent to 90 percent of human diseases.[25]
- Chemicals in our environment have been connected to ovarian cancer, prostate cancer, breast cancer, early onset of menopause, diminished sperm quality, fertility difficulties, and heart disease, obesity, and diabetes.[26] (And that's the short list.)
- People who get 17 to 21 percent of their calories from added sugar have a 38 percent higher risk of dying from cardiovascular disease than those who get 8 percent of their calories from sugar.[27] Studies have also linked a higher sugar intake—especially from sugar-sweetened beverages—to a higher risk of developing autoimmune diseases like rheumatoid arthritis.[28]
- As little as fifteen minutes of physical activity a day can boost your life-span by three years; other studies have shown that exercising can help reduce allergic inflammation.[29]

These are just a few examples of the huge impact your lifestyle and environment have on how well you feel each day. In fact, they may even be more important than your genetic predispositions. In recent years, a now-popular field of study has developed called epigenetics, which investigates how our environment and behavior can turn different genes on and off. Epigenetics (which roughly translates to the subject of factors "above the gene") teaches us that it's possible, through lifestyle change, to change how our DNA expresses itself. These modifications can influence how cells divide and what proteins are made, and even what genetic material is passed on to our offspring. (Yes, the effects of an unhealthy lifestyle can be passed down to your kids!) We're all born with DNA that isn't going to change, but epigenetics tells us that lifestyle factors really make the difference between your developing a chronic disease and not. This is great news. It means that even if you have a genetic predisposition to a certain disease—say, obesity or breast cancer or Alzheimer's—you have a *lot* of control over whether you develop that disease. When you can tweak your environment, you can literally change how your genes express themselves and get your immune health back on track.

TAKING THE IMMUNE DYSFUNCTION CRISIS HEAD-ON

Admittedly, there are plenty of books out there that teach you how to get healthy and prevent chronic disease. But here's where those books fail: They tend to forget that the root cause of the disease is different for different people, and that diseases almost always tie back to the immune system. Many books will prescribe one lifestyle technique (e.g., yoga, meditation, or fasting) or one diet (e.g., low-fat, ketogenic, Paleolithic, grain-free, or Mediterranean) as the cure-all for disease and the perfect change for everyone's best health. And while each of these has salient points and research to back them up, they are not absolutely right or wrong for each person. Thanks to our different Immunotypes, some of us thrive following a lifestyle or nutrition plan that others might suffer from.

In this book, we're taking a more refined and individualized approach. In the following pages I will teach you exactly how to make specific changes in your habits, environment, and diet, as well as use focused natural treatments to nudge your immune system back into balance. This will help you restore healthy inflammation levels and develop a healthier relationship with the microbes in the environment—and make sure that your environment is leading to the optimal expression of your genes.

I make such a big deal out of achieving immune system health because our immune systems can be lifesaving when they're working properly and both wildly ineffective and incredibly destructive when they're not. There are cells in our immune system that are more powerful than any man-made drug in the world. For example, some cells can inject bacteria with chemicals and blow them up; others can identify and swallow harmful parasites whole. And yet, in other situations, these same cells can reject transplanted organs, destroy our own red blood cells, or put us into anaphylactic shock. Seriously impressive for a bunch of cells that we can't see with the naked eye, isn't it? Our immune system has a lot on its plate. Every single day it monitors everything that's touching our skin, floating up through our nose, and going down our throats. We encounter about 100 million viruses and bacteria daily that we need to prevent from infecting our body, so our immune system revs up, gets into an inflammatory state, kills what it needs to kill, and then resolves before we even notice.

One of the major reasons why the immune dysfunction crisis has gotten so bad is because attaining an in-depth understanding of the complex workings of your immune system can take years. Much as with our hormones or our brains, there's just so much left to learn about how the immune system works. That said, in the last few decades we've learned a *lot* about all the moving pieces of the immune system, how they fit together, and what role they play in keeping us healthy. Having a basic understanding of the immune system is critical to reestablishing balance, so in the next chapter, we're headed to the classroom.

CHAPTER 2

Immunity 101—Understanding Your Immune Army

Remember when I said that the human immune system is an enigma to much of the medical community? And that it's composed of endless cells, receptors, and messengers that can make even the smartest head spin? Well, I wasn't lying. You can study the intricacies of the immune system for years and still end up scratching your head while reading a new study or report. But it's important to take on the challenge, because having a basic understanding of the immune system is critical. We learned this lesson with the COVID-19 pandemic when many of us were set back on our heels, lacking the knowledge and confidence to understand the severity of the threat, calculate our own risk, and make decisions that would help us protect ourselves. Many of us felt overwhelmed, underprepared, and like we had a lot of catching up to do.

But here's the good news: You only need the CliffsNotes version of the immune system to grasp the concepts of what's driving your Immunotype and make a plan to get your immune system back in balance. This chapter will set the stage so you can appreciate how your immune system works on a day-to-day basis and what happens when it veers toward being Smoldering, Misguided, Hyperactive, or Weak. I'm going to be introducing quite a few concepts here that you may never have heard of, so bear with me! I've tried to focus on giving you the information you *really* need, without getting so far into the nitty-gritty that you end up throwing this book against the wall.

YOUR VERY OWN IMMUNE ARMY

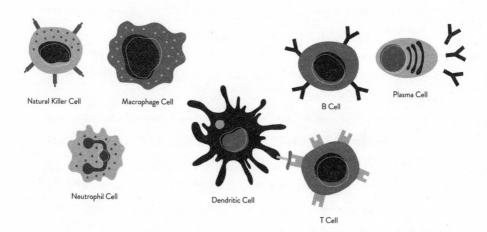

Natural Killer Cell

Macrophage Cell

Plasma Cell

B Cell

Neutrophil Cell

Dendritic Cell

T Cell

There are a ton of analogies to choose from when it comes to the immune system, but the one I find most fitting is to describe it as if it were an army—your own personal army that lives inside your body! We have no choice but to interact with the outside world and face threats of injury and disease (not unless we're willing to live in a bubble), and therefore, we need a built-in system to battle threats to our health. This system has to be swift, smart, and efficient, which means there need to be a lot of active fighters that work together toward the common goal of protecting you— hence the army analogy.

When you're born, your army is immature and you mostly rely on the antibodies passed from your mother and contained in breast-milk to protect you from infections. As we've already learned, you get your first inoculation of friendly microbes during your first moments on earth. This means that in your first few days, your immune system army is already starting to recruit soldiers and begin training. And just as the army is divided into branches, your immune system is too. The two main branches are called the "innate immune system" and the "adaptive immune system." Each branch has different goals and its own unique soldiers, weapons, and communication systems, but they also work together to optimize protection.

We'll start with the innate immune system, which is composed of the soldiers on the front line of the metaphorical immune system battlefield.

THE INNATE IMMUNE SYSTEM: THE FRONTLINE SOLDIERS

Let's suppose you're out for a jog when you trip over a curb and fall, leaving a big gash on your knee. In a split second, bacteria from the dirty street manage to catch a ride into your body through your broken skin. Yuck, right? Lucky for you, there's a multitude of innate immune system cells that patrol your body at all hours of the day and night, working to recognize particular patterns and signals that are common to many bacteria, viruses, fungi, and other invaders.

The innate immune system is responsible for our "nonspecific immunity," which means it launches a general protective response to an antigen, which is a molecule on the surface of most invaders that the immune system can recognize. The word "innate" means "inborn" or "natural," so it shouldn't come as a surprise that the innate immune system is the part of the immune system we're born with, not the part of the immune system that evolves in response to different germs we encounter throughout our lifetime. The innate immune system tends to get weaker as we age. In fact, it's why older people are at higher risk of severe COVID-19, while children aren't nearly as affected.

The innate immune system is our first line of defense against all invaders and injury and includes the physical and physiological barriers that help keep harmful substances out of our bodies in the first place. Components of our innate immune system include:

- Our cough reflex, which helps us expel things that may irritate or infect us.
- The various enzymes in tears and skin oils.
- Mucus production, which traps bacteria and small particles and helps expel them from the body.
- Our skin, which acts as a physical barrier between our inner world and the outside world.
- Our stomach acid, which helps kill microbes that enter through our food and water.

The innate immune system is also composed of cells that are trained to respond to the common molecules or antigens found in many foreign substances, including bacteria, viruses, and parasites. You can think of these cells as soldiers that are stationed in different places throughout the body, constantly patrolling for potential threats. The strength of the immune system lies in its ability to respond extremely quickly to foreign microbes and to prevent them from spreading throughout the body until the more specialized cells can arrive at the scene. So, when that nasty bacterium from the street gets into your bloodstream through an open cut, your innate immune system recognizes it and sounds the alarm, waking up a whole posse of defenders.

THE INNATE IMMUNE SOLDIERS: PHAGOCYTES, NK CELLS, AND NEUTROPHILS

Some of the most crucial soldiers of the innate immune army are called "professional phagocytes." Because I'm a child of the 1980s, I like to think of these as the Pac-Men (or Pac-Women) of the immune system. They love to gobble things up. "Phago" means "to eat" in Greek, and "cyte" means "cell." So basically, these cells are professional eaters. (Not a bad job to have, right?!) The most important types of phagocytes are macrophages, neutrophils, and dendritic cells. As you can probably guess from the name, macrophages are just really large phagocytes. They hang out in tissues like your skin, lungs, and intestines, and scan for dangerous invaders they can gobble up. When they're not busy eating invaders, they act as the garbage collectors of the immune system, cleaning up cellular debris to keep your body in tip-top shape. When things start to get a little overwhelming for a macrophage, it can communicate to other cells of the immune system (through a series of complex chemical messengers that we'll learn about soon) that it needs backup. That's where neutrophils step in. These cells are sort of like the kamikaze pilots of the immune system; in other words, they're "born to die," but not before they do some serious damage. When neutrophils roll up to the scene, they ingest pathogens and inject them with toxic chemicals, literally liquefying them at the sight of infection. (Fun fact: This is what causes pus—the thick yellowish or greenish liquid that appears when you have an infection.) The downside of this chemical soup is that it can also inflict injury upon your tissues, leading to a lot of collateral damage. A little bit of this is okay, but if the mess that neutrophils make doesn't get resolved quickly enough and there continues to be a source of infection, this cycle of toxic soup can persist and create serious damage and chronic inflammation.

Another big soldier in our innate immune lineup is the aptly named "natural killer cell," abbreviated as "NK cell." This guy is a powerful weapon in our war against many types of infections, but its specialty is viruses. In fact, if you have a genetic deficiency of NK cells, you will likely have problems keeping certain viruses under control, such as those that cause cold sores or warts caused by herpes simplex virus and human papillomavirus. NK cells are also our primary ammunition for identifying cancer cells and destroying them before they can replicate and spread. NK cells are lethal, and they inject enzymes into virally infected or cancerous cells, instructing them to "commit suicide."

We couldn't wrap up our discussion of the innate immune system without talking about one of the most interesting soldiers—the star-shaped "dendritic cell." Dendritic cells act as a sort of courier between our innate immune system and the other branch of our immune system, the adaptive immune system. Dendritic cells work similarly to macrophages in that they can sample and engulf bits of invaders, but then instead of gobbling them up altogether, they hurry off and present them to the cells of our adaptive immune system so that more specialized cells can make an educated decision about what to do next. Dendritic cells tend to hang out at the border between our internal world and the outside, constantly patrolling our skin, nose, lungs, and GI tract.

As you can see, our innate immune system has a lot of different soldiers cruising around our bodies 24/7, working together to kill dangerous invaders and cancer cells, and then cleaning up the mess afterward. It seems like a lot of complicated logistics, doesn't it? It is! Luckily, our immune system has a highly sophisticated communications network. This is really the secret sauce of our immunity. Without it, our immune system would just be a bunch of cells bumbling around without any marching orders.

THE WONDERFUL WORLD OF CYTOKINES

Could you imagine if the entire system of cell towers, landlines, digital networks, and mail services went down in this country? I shudder to think about what kind of predicament we'd be in. Without any communication, our society as we know it would collapse. Well, that's how crucial our cytokine system is to our immune function. In fact, 5G has nothing on our cytokines.

There are well over a hundred known cytokine chemicals that act as messengers between our immune cells. All of our immune cells secrete and receive different cytokine messages using receptors on their surfaces, sort of like little cell towers or Wi-Fi routers. Cytokines often get a bad rap because of their role in causing big inflammatory problems such as "cytokine storms," transplant rejection, and septic shock, but when you zoom out on cytokines, you'll see that maligning them entirely is unfair and an example of how oversimplifying systems in the body can lead us astray. Why? Because there are plenty of inflammatory, regulatory, and anti-inflammatory cytokines doing their jobs every day keeping you alive, healthy, and in balance. They're all necessary.

So what are cytokines, and how many are there? You'd go cross-eyed if I listed all the cytokines in your body (there are multiple types of cytokines, and different families within each type, leading to more than a hundred confusing names and symbols).

The good news is that it's not necessary to memorize every single one. To appreciate how your personal Immunotype forms and how you can change it, you just need to grasp a little of the parlance. Just know that when cytokines are signaling properly, they're a huge asset to your immune system; but when the signaling goes awry, they can be major contributors to immune issues and the development of the four Immunotypes. So get a strong cup of coffee and bear with me for a few minutes. These are some of the major families of cytokines that we need to be familiar with.

1. Interleukins (ILs)

There are about forty of these chemicals, and each plays a huge role in fighting infections of all kinds, as well as calming down the immune response. One of their most famous roles is to cause a fever, which helps raise the body temperature to fight off microbes. Interleukins are secreted by many different cells of both our innate and our adaptive immune system. In appropriate numbers they're a good thing, but when they spin out of control, ILs are often responsible for chronic inflammation and allergies, which makes them relevant to more than one Immunotype.

2. Interferons (IFNs)

These bad boys are the key to defending against viruses and tumors. They come in three basic flavors—alpha (α), beta (β), and gamma (γ)—and they earned their name from their ability to "interfere" with reproducing viruses and cancer cells. You can think of them as an SOS signal, because IFNs are secreted from virally infected cells and cancer cells as a cry for help. They signal to other cells like NK cells and macrophages to come kill the bad guys. They are also partially responsible for the fevers and body aches you get when you're sick. Interferon therapy is helpful in treating cancer and hepatitis, and certain interferon blockers are used to treat autoimmune diseases such as multiple sclerosis and rheumatoid arthritis, which occur when IFN signaling is misguided.

3. Tumor Necrosis Factor (TNF)

As the name suggests, this chemical is involved in helping to degrade cancer cells, but it also works against viruses and bacteria. TNF gets secreted from macrophages to help recruit other cells like neutrophils and natural killer cells to join the battle when an infection is present. TNF is also a key cytokine secreted from certain types of T cells (which are one of the main cell types of the adaptive immune system that we'll learn about in a minute) to keep up the inflammatory fight against invaders and bacteria. When TNF is not signaling correctly, it can be a big player in the tissue destruction seen in several autoimmune diseases; in fact, drugs for diseases like Crohn's disease and rheumatoid arthritis often block TNF from signaling.

Whew! That's it. That wasn't too bad, was it? Later on, when we get to talk about your specific Immunotype, you'll gain an even deeper understanding of how lifestyle factors influence the cytokine signaling system, for better or for worse!

YOUR ADAPTIVE IMMUNE RESPONSE: THE SPECIAL OPS TEAM

Our innate immune system is pretty awesome in defending us against all matter of antigens. It can jump into action the second a threat is detected, but sometimes, that's not enough. Bacteria and viruses are pretty wily organisms; they can evade defenses and mutate into more resistant pathogens that can trick and overwhelm our innate immune system. When this happens, the soldiers of our innate immune system need to call for backup. Luckily, we have a masterful set of cells that can jump into gear to adapt to these challenges, identify invaders in a way that is more specific, and create memory cells to protect us when an antigen shows up again, even if it's years or decades later. Liken this to a soldier who's trying to take down his target but then realizes he's in over his head. Instead, he calls for backup, and fellow soldiers who are trained in special ops come in to save the day. These high-level soldiers are your adaptive immune cells, which are responsible for "acquired" or "antigen-specific" immunity.

B CELLS AND T CELLS: THE SOLDIERS OF YOUR ADAPTIVE IMMUNE RESPONSE

The main thing to know about the adaptive immune response is that it's specific to the antigen and is acquired over the course of our lifetime as we're exposed to more and more germs (hence the labels "acquired immunity" and "antigen-specific immunity"). Our adaptive immune system has memory, which explains why we don't get the same infection twice, and is also responsible for the effectiveness of vaccines. The adaptive immune response is also what helps us distinguish between our body's own tissues and foreign invaders, which means it's critical for preventing autoimmune disease. Essential to these activities are the two main cells of the adaptive immune system, called lymphocytes: B cells and T cells.

B Cells and Antibodies: Our Body's Data Collectors

B cells are remarkable for two big reasons. First, they have a great memory, and second, they can make antibodies, which are proteins produced in response to a specific antigen on a virus or bacteria that provide us with immunity to the illness caused by that specific infection. In their infancy, B cells have the potential to recognize hundreds of thousands of different viruses and bacteria, but until they come in contact with a specific one, they're inactive and just hang out in our lymph nodes. But once a B cell comes into contact with an antigen, usually on the surface of an infected cell or bacteria, it moves out of the lymph nodes into the bloodstream. Once there, it transforms into one of two things: (1) a different type of B cell called a "plasma B cell" that goes on to generate gobs of antibodies against the antigen; or (2) a "memory B cell," which will stay in your body for years so that when you come into contact with the antigen again, that memory cell will be able to rapidly defend you. As you might already have guessed, both plasma and memory B cells are why vaccines create long-term protective immunity and why, as in the case of chicken pox or mononucleosis, we don't usually fall ill to the same infection twice.

As we just learned, one of the main jobs of plasma B cells is to make antibodies, also called immunoglobulins. Antibodies work by recognizing specific invaders, grabbing them, and marking them for destruction by other immune cells. There are several "classes" of antibodies, which look and act differently. The most important immunoglobulins are IgM, IgG, IgA, and IgE. IgM is our "early defense" antibody against antigens. It's highly effective at tagging invaders for destruction by other cells, but it has a short life-span. So after IgM is produced, B cells switch over to IgG production, which gives us longer-term protection against an antigen. These IgG antibodies can linger for years or even a lifetime. IgA antibodies are the antibodies we have the most of, and that's because they have to cover all of our mucosal surfaces, like our mouth, lungs, sinuses, and GI tract. They don't float around much in our bloodstream but stay fixed in place. Like a bouncer at a bar, IgA plays a huge role in protecting our body from unwanted invaders—especially viruses. Lastly, IgE is our "allergic antibody." IgE is really there to protect us from invasion by parasites—it can identify and mark these nasty worms and amoebas so that other cells can take them down. But when it's out of balance, IgE orchestrates the release of histamine and chemicals that give us annoying seasonal sneezing, runny nose, asthma, and food allergies.

If you're thinking "Wow, B cells seem pretty important," you are correct! They're very important. And while it sounds like they've thought of everything, B cells don't and can't run the adaptive immune system all on their own. They have lots of help from that wonderful cytokine messaging system we just learned about. Cytokine signaling is what helps B cells understand that they need to make IgG to fight strep throat, or IgA to kill the rotavirus your kid brought home from day care, or IgE to destroy that parasite you picked up on your yoga retreat in India. B cells also require the help of the other main cells of the adaptive immune system: T cells, which, as you'll learn, are one of the major underlying influences in the four Immunotypes, determining whether we have allergies, whether we can mount effective responses to bacteria and viruses, and even whether or not we develop an inflammatory or autoimmune disease.

T Cells: The Generals of Our Immune System

As amazing as B cells and their wonderful antibodies are, the real power of the adaptive immune system lies with our T cells—the kingpin cells. There are two main types of T cells—the "helper T cell" and the "killer T cell." The illustrious and multitalented helper T cell is the true mastermind behind our immune response, something that was demonstrated with devastating consequences during the AIDS epidemic of the 1980s. How? Because the HIV virus specifically attacks helper T cells and destroys them, resulting in severe immune deficiency that caused HIV-positive patients to die from illnesses that would normally be no big deal. Since the 1980s, we've learned a lot about how helper T cells are like the data scientists of our immune system. They receive messages from our innate immune system cells, like the macrophages and dendritic cells we learned about earlier, and they can translate this information so that our body can understand what it's up against. The helper T cells answer questions like: What are we dealing with? Is it a fungus, parasite, bacteria, or virus? Where in the body is the problem located? Which immune cells need to be alerted?

Once the T cells have this information, things get really cool. Depending on the type of invader you're dealing with, a custom subtype of helper T cell is made to take it on. Before a T cell comes in contact with any pathogens, it is "naïve," but once it knows what it's up against, it transforms into a specific helper T cell. This whole process allows our immune system to be precise and effective in clearing out infections and repairing inflammation. The prevalence of these specific subtypes of helper T cells also plays a central role in creating the four different Immunotypes. Why? Because once our body starts producing these different types of T cells, they can sometimes get stuck in a pattern

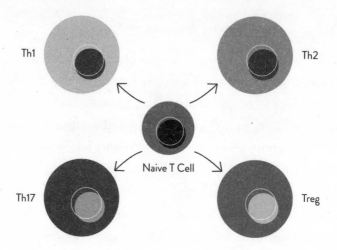

where they start producing too much of the same type, leading to an imbalance. The four main subtype helper T cells are Th1, Th2, Th17, and regulatory; too much of any of them can alter your immune response and lead to different symptoms and diseases.

To make matters worse, once helper T cells have committed to their career as either TH1, TH2, TH17, or regulatory T cells, they can't change back. They start to pump out cytokines that prompt their own kind to proliferate, creating a snowball effect. If we don't get unstuck, this imbalance or dominance in subtype helper T cells—which is also called "T cell polarization"—can affect cytokine signaling, leading to a Smoldering, Misguided, Hyperactive, or Weak Immunotype.

The other type of T cell to note is the killer T cell. These cells are able to destroy infected cells directly, similarly to the natural killer cells of our innate immune system. The selling point of killer T cells is their ability to recognize a *specific* invader—such as a virus, a cancer cell, or a cell that is damaged in some way—and then destroy it all on its own. Killer T cells are extremely helpful in the right context, but when they get knocked out of balance, it spells trouble for your body. In fact, killer T cells have been implicated in the progression of multiple diseases. For example, in juvenile (type 1) diabetes, killer T cells destroy insulin-producing cells in the pancreas, and in rheumatoid arthritis, killer T cells damage joint tissue.[1] However, without killer T cells, we wouldn't be able to fight viruses like the Epstein-Barr virus (EBV).[2] See, again, how it's all about balance?

As we move into the Immune Restoration Plan, one of our main focuses will be supporting healthy T cell balance, especially when it comes to helper T cells. And here's where the good news comes in: Most helper T cells and their subtypes don't live that long after they've done their job, so there's ample opportunity to reverse that snowball effect and get back on the right track. We'll do that by changing several lifestyle factors: our sleep, stress, gut health, environmental, and nutritional habits. By making these specific shifts, we can target the behavior of T cells in a way that shifts our imbalanced Immunotype back to one that's healthy and strong.

YOUR IMMUNE SYSTEM ARMY GLOSSARY

Phew! You made it. Congratulations, you are now your very own immune system expert. I threw a lot at you in this chapter, so if you don't remember everything—don't worry! I've created a glossary of the terms we just learned, and I recommend earmarking this page and coming back to it anytime you encounter a word or name that you don't remember. Especially when we start talking about lifestyle changes, I'll be citing research that measures factors like helper T cells, antibodies, and specific cytokines, so it'll be helpful to have a quick reference guide.

1. **Antigens:** Antigens are molecules or structures found both in and on the surface of cells that can be recognized by our immune system. They are found on outside invaders but also on our own cells, food molecules, and toxins. They by definition can elicit an antibody response.

2. **Innate immune system:** The innate immune system is our body's first line of defense, responding immediately to slow the spread of damage or infection. It creates "nonspecific" immunity, and we're born with it.

3. **Phagocytes:** Think of phagocytes as being the Pac-Men of the immune system. They are professional eaters that engulf microbes as well as damaged cells. There are three main types:
   - **Macrophages:** Macrophages are large phagocytes that hang out in your tissues, scanning for dangerous invaders that they can gobble up. They also clean up cellular debris, acting as the "garbage collectors" of the immune system.
   - **Neutrophils:** Neutrophils are a type of phagocyte that ingests pathogens, but they also inject a soup of toxic chemicals into the invader, which creates toxic debris that needs to be cleaned up.
   - **Dendritic cells:** These star-shaped cells act as couriers between our innate and adaptive immune systems, sampling bits of invaders and then presenting them to our B cells and T cells.

4. **Natural killer cells (NK cells):** These innate immune cells inject lethal enzymes into virally infected or cancerous cells, instructing them to die.

5. **Cytokines:** Cytokines are the chemical messengers for both the innate and the adaptive immune system. Some commonly mentioned cytokines are tumor necrosis factor (TNF), interferons (IFNs), and interleukins (ILs). Cytokine signaling issues can

become underlying causes of the imbalances in the immune system that we see with the four Immunotypes.

6. **Adaptive immune system:** The adaptive immune system is in charge of our "antigen-specific" or "acquired" immune response, which is established over the course of our lifetimes.

7. **B cells:** These are adaptive immune cells that create memory and make antibodies that are specific to an antigen.

   - **Plasma B cells:** These B cells make antibodies.
   - **Memory B cells:** These B cells create memories of specific antigens to offer you long-term protection.

8. **Antibodies:** These are proteins made by plasma B cells that are able to lock onto the surface of an invading cell and mark it for destruction by other immune cells.

9. **T cells:** These adaptive immune cells multiply and differentiate into helper or killer T cells.

   - **Helper T cell:** Helper T cells stimulate B cells to make antibodies, affect cytokine signaling, and help killer T cells develop. There are four main types of helper T cells: TH1, TH2, TH17, and regulatory T cells.
   - **Killer T cell:** Activated by cytokines, killer T cells directly bind to and kill cells that have already been infected by a foreign invader.

Now that we understand the immune dysfunction crisis and have a basic understanding of the major players in the immune system, it's time to dive even deeper into what, exactly, goes wrong with our immune systems to create the four Immunotypes. The answer to that question is the buzzword everyone seems to be talking about—*inflammation*. What causes chronic inflammation, what triggers it in the first place, and is there anything we can really do about it? These questions and more will be answered in the next chapter.

CHAPTER 3

Chronic Inflammation—The Heart of Immune System Imbalance

How do you spot chronic inflammation? Do you need special X-ray vision? Chronic inflammation cloaks itself in many disguises that I see every day. I see it in my patient Greg, who has high blood pressure and keeps gaining weight, and also Bill, because he's sick and stressed all the time. It's also in Kelly, whose asthma is flaring up, and Rachel when her arthritis is out of control. On the surface, these all look so different, but pull back the curtain and you'll see one thing they have in common—chronic inflammation. This is the root issue that leads to imbalanced Immunotypes and eventually to all of our medical woes. These imbalances don't just spring up overnight. They're the result of years and sometimes decades of exposures, stressors, and other factors that eventually culminate in getting diagnosed one day with an illness or disease. That's why in this chapter, we'll be taking a deeper look at inflammation and how it contributes to all four Immunotypes.

INFLAMMATION — CAN'T LIVE WITH IT, CAN'T LIVE WITHOUT IT

Rubor, calor, dolar, and *tumor* are the Latin words the first-century roman scholar Aulus Cornelius Celsus used to describe inflammation.[1] And while we know a heck of a lot more about inflammation than we did two thousand years ago, "redness, heat, pain, and swelling" are still accurate descriptions of what we all experience when we get inflamed. Admittedly, those four things don't sound like much fun. And if you've read anything about inflammation in the news, blogs, or other books, you might be under the impression that it's all bad and your life depends on stamping it out completely. "Anti-inflammatory" has become synonymous with "healthy" in many circles.

Well, that's only half true. Here's a more accurate description: Inflammation is an absolutely necessary part of being alive; it's an integral part of our immune system activation and protects us from harm of all sorts.

The lifesaving inflammatory response looks like this: Let's say you sprain your ankle and within a few hours, it's swollen like a red balloon, bruised, and painful, and you can't walk on it. Hooray! This is your immune system in action, opening up blood vessels to bring fluid, blood, and white blood cells to correct the tissue damage and heal the injury so you can be off your crutches in a few days. The same thing happens when you get strep throat. You have swollen lymph nodes, a fiery red throat, fever, and pus on your tonsils, which all resolve in a week or so. In the first case, injured ligaments and muscles activate our inflammatory response, and the response is to knit up and heal the damage caused by the sprain. In the case of strep throat and other infections, your body is trying to defend against dangerous foreign microbes, so the inflammatory response here is focused on killing. Without a speedy inflammatory response, you'd be miserably sick constantly. Viruses, bacteria, and other infections would lead to severe illness almost all of the time, and it would take us forever to recover from injuries and surgeries. So be happy that you can get inflamed in the first place! After an infection or injury clears up, however, there's often collateral damage, so the second part of a healthy inflammatory response is resolution and cleaning up the mess. *This is often where things start to go wrong.*

WHEN INFLAMMATION HURTS INSTEAD OF HELPS

The immune system's central task is to keep us alive and healthy by seeking out and destroying dangerous bacteria, viruses, parasites, and cancer cells. To do this, we must become inflamed in the short term, kill these unwanted invaders, and then reverse course quickly to clear out and repair the damage. The process is much like a controlled burn in a forest fire—the soil, forest, and weather conditions need to be perfect, allowing effective burning without igniting a raging inferno. The immune system needs a well-trained fire brigade to carry out its job without a spillover effect.

Unfortunately, this doesn't always go as planned. When we have damaged tissue or infectious microbes in our body, cells in the area start sending up flares for help in the form of cytokines. This is the battle cry for immune cells like neutrophils to come to the area to gobble up microbes and engulf damaged tissues. As I said earlier, neutrophils die after they've done their work of killing. This is called "apoptosis," or programmed cell death. Apoptosis is a very tidy and organized death that takes a few hours and happens to all cells of our body, not just our immune cells. In fact, when cells are made to die they set an internal timer like a ticking time bomb that goes off and then signals macrophages (remember, these are the Pac-Men and garbage collectors of the immune system!) to rush in and eat the whole cell and its contents without leaving a mess. This process even sends out additional anti-inflammatory signals to calm down inflammation in the aftermath of the threat. (I've always thought it was pretty amazing that the last dying effort of the neutrophil was to tell the body "Everything is okay now.")

But what happens when there aren't enough macrophages around to fully clean up and resolve the mess? The neutrophils full of dead microbes wait around like a stinky garbage can on trash day. And when they aren't gobbled up, they start to leak out their toxic contents, which only causes more damage, stimulates more inflammatory cytokine messengers, and attracts more neutrophils to the area, requiring more macrophages to pick up the trash. As you can see, a messy cycle ensues of cell death, inadequate cleanup, more cell death, and more cleanup. This nonresolving inflammation is one of the key issues underlying many diseases. In fact, failure to remove these dead neutrophils is a major underlying cause of autoimmune disease.

Another way that we stay inflamed is thanks to a malfunctioning danger signal that won't shut off. Here's what I mean by that: Inside all of our cells, we have a group of danger-sensing proteins that are collectively called NLRP. These proteins can sense when our cells get infected with a microbe or get damaged by a toxin and are even able to sense when there are damaged and dying cells nearby. Like a self-destructive Trojan horse, these NLRP proteins join inside the cell and form a structure called an inflammasome, which directs the cell to self-destruct in a fiery death called "pyroptosis." It does this to prevent the spread of infections that cannot live outside the cell, like viruses, but it also sends out superinflammatory cytokines like interleukin-1 beta (IL-1β) to alert the rest of the immune system to a nearby threat. This happens on a regular basis, and normally, things can return to balance pretty quickly, but sometimes this danger signal and this inflammasome activity get stuck in the on position and many cells start to go up in flames, sending danger signals to their neighbor cells and encouraging them to jump ship and do the same. Chronic viral infections and toxins can signal this inflammasome activity, but so can damaged tissue in our heart vessels, uric acid crystals found in gout-ridden joints, and even plaques found in the brains of Alzheimer's patients. As you can see, this is another way that chronic inflammation in the body can cause even more inflammation and cell death; it's also another example of how working on removing sources of chronic inflammation, which we'll learn about a little later, can help our immune system become healthier by preventing this ongoing cycle of our inflammasomes getting out of control.

Lastly, another inflammation promoter is a protein that we have in all of our cells called NF-κB (nuclear factor kappa B). This protein floats around inside our cells, waiting for a signal like damaged cells, viruses, toxins, inflammatory cytokines, or really any triggers to show up. When that signal finally arrives, it activates NF-κB to transcribe our DNA, turning on genes to make proteins. This doesn't sound bad, but the purpose of these proteins is to activate immune cells and cytokines, ramping up inflammation. If you're thinking, "Wow, this is getting a little too complicated for me...," I totally get it. Why do I even tell you about inflammasomes, NF-κB, and fiery cell death when you didn't sign up for a college-level immunology class? Because I want you to understand your inflammation targets. Like the great Chinese general Sun Tzu said: "Know your enemies and know yourself and you will not be imperiled in a hundred battles."

When we can visualize how unhealthy lifestyle choices turn these inflammation switches on—and how healthy lifestyle choices turn them off—it makes it that much easier to reach for the piece of fresh fruit instead of the candy bar. After all, instead of just wondering if the turmeric tea you're drinking at night is helping inflammation, wouldn't it be better to *know* that with every sip you're shutting down that NF-κB system and making small steps toward a less-inflamed future? Knowledge is power.

CYTOKINE STORMS AND A DISTRACTED IMMUNE SYSTEM

We just learned some pretty complicated mechanisms behind an unhealthy inflammatory response. To review, a rogue immune response typically occurs for three main reasons:

- Inflammation is triggered when it's not needed.
- Inflammation is not resolving.
- The original source of the inflammation isn't going away.

Now, the next logical question is: What can we do about it? You might feel like the inflammatory response exists so deep in your body that you have no control over it. But you'd be wrong! In fact, when we need to decrease chronic inflammation to bring balance back to our immune system, our first order of business should be to double down on finding the sources of *unnecessary inflammation in our life*. It'll come as no surprise that this is also a big part of the Immune Restoration Plan.

The best way I can explain this is that our bodies are smart, but sometimes we can be...well, not so smart. As humans, we constantly introduce things to our body that make it inflamed, causing the immune system to get distracted from the more important job of protecting us from dangerous invaders. These distractions might be indulging in excess sugar, skimping on sleep, overexercising, being sedentary, or drinking too much alcohol—really anything that damages our tissues or stresses our body. It's like constantly checking your email and social media feeds when you should be focusing on that important deadline for work. When we have nonproductive inflammation throughout the body in response to all these inflammatory triggers, it dilutes our immune power and makes us more vulnerable to everyday threats that would normally be no big deal.

This truth has been exemplified in the COVID-19 pandemic. We saw that diseases like diabetes and heart disease, as well as old age, were risk factors for poor outcomes for SARS CoV-2. The chronic inflammation from these states weakens the innate immune system and allows the virus to enter and spread throughout the body relatively undetected. In the case of "cytokine storms," the adaptive immune system takes over and, in a desperate last attempt to protect the body, starts to pump out inflammatory cytokines all over the body in a way that's totally out of control. This "cytokine storm" massively damages our cells, triggering a hectic repair response that can't keep up with the damage, and we end up in septic shock with a grim prognosis. By removing unnecessary chronic inflammation, we can make sure the immune system is ready for a threat and prevent deadly outcomes like this.

GETTING TO THE ROOT OF INFLAMMATION

The inner workings of the immune system and the inflammatory response are endlessly complicated, but the truth is that the causes

of chronic inflammation are pretty simple. And even better—
they're almost totally within your control. That means that by making
the changes we will discuss throughout this book, you'll be able
to give your immune system a leg up and minimize your risk for
chronic inflammation and a distracted immune system.

The biggest source of nonproductive inflammation in our
lives comes from what we decide to put in our mouths. Every day
you make choices about what's at the end of your fork, and
some of these decisions cause inflammation, while others reduce
it. When it comes to food, the biggest sources of inflammation
are:

- **Unhealthy oils:** Foods that are higher in certain types of
  fats, like polyunsaturated industrial seed oils such as soy-
  bean oil, canola oil (rapeseed oil), sunflower oil, corn oil,
  cottonseed oil, "vegetable" oil, safflower oil, peanut oil, and
  grapeseed oil, should all be avoided. For years we were told
  to consume more of these polyunsaturated omega-6–rich
  vegetable oils, but more recent data has shown them to be
  highly unstable and linked to inflammatory diseases.[2] Instead
  we should focus on healthy fats from whole foods such as
  nuts and seeds, olive oil, organic coconut oil, and wild-
  caught fish. And although saturated fat was demonized for
  years as a major cause of heart disease, as it can increase total
  cholesterol in some people, we now know that some saturated fats—whether from coconuts or eggs—can be part of
  a healthy diet as long as they come from a high-quality
  organic source and are not eaten in excess.
- **Trans fats:** Trans fats should be avoided like the plague.
  These fats are liquid oils that are synthesized into solid fats
  and are found in shortening like Crisco, margarine, and
  many snack food items like crackers, cookies, pizza, fast

food, and even peanut butter! Trans fats elevate LDL cholesterol and insulin and lower beneficial HDL cholesterol. They're associated with an increase in many diseases, such as heart disease, obesity, colon cancer, and diabetes.[3]

- **Sugar:** Hands down, if you want to do one thing to lower inflammation in your body, I would recommend taking out as many forms of excess sugar in your diet as possible. This includes the obvious, like high-fructose corn syrup and the sucrose found in candy, soda, and baked goods, but also some so-called health foods that contain obscene amounts of sugar, like granolas, protein bars, yogurts, vegan and gluten-free baked goods, and juices. Studies have linked a high intake of added sugar to increased heart disease, obesity, diabetes, and fatty liver disease.[4][5][6] Even refined carbohydrates like pasta, white flour, bread, and other starches will turn into excess glucose in the body and drive up inflammation. This doesn't mean that you should go super-low-carb, which comes with its own set of problems for your mood, sleep, and energy levels. The golden rule is to focus on fiber-rich, whole-plant carbohydrates—like those in vegetables, fruits, legumes, and whole grains—instead of simple, refined carbohydrates.

- **Too much alcohol:** Yes, I know, what about the French paradox and the fact that drinking red wine is good for you? Actually, that didn't really pan out. Turns out that alcohol has multiple deleterious effects on our immune system, including weakening our gut-immune barrier, damaging our microbiome, and causing significant oxidative stress on our cells.[7] Once broken down in the liver, ethanol creates toxins that over time increase your risk of cancer and premature aging. When you think about it, that sort of takes the fun out of it, doesn't it? Overall, alcohol should be minimized, and despite much industry-driven data on its benefits, that data really hasn't been shown to be true.

It's not just food that contributes to chronic inflammation, either. Here are some other big instigators of inflammation:

- **Excess body fat:** A critical part of fighting inflammation is keeping your body composition in a healthy place. This may go without saying, but excess fat on your body—especially around your midsection—makes you inflamed. In fact, visceral body fat acts like its own organ, secreting a whole host of inflammatory cytokines, setting you up for metabolic syndrome.[8]
- **Tobacco:** This should be a no-brainer, but even the chemicals in second- and even thirdhand smoke are carcinogens. The damage that these products create in our tissues keeps us inflamed and in a constant state of repair.
- **Stress:** Chronic, unmanaged emotional and physical stress elevates inflammatory cytokine release, and people who have high physical and emotional stressors have greater levels of inflammation. In fact, C-reactive protein (CRP), which is a marker for inflammation, goes up in patients under acute stress.[9]
- **Lack of sleep:** Skimping on sleep or sleeping poorly is a huge factor driving inflammation, which is one of the reasons why sleep deprivation is a major contributor to chronic metabolic diseases like diabetes, obesity, heart disease, and stroke.
- **Sitting too much:** Sitting is the new smoking. Humans were made to move, but given our modern lifestyles—commuting to work, sitting at a desk, and being glued to our screens—we've become supersedentary. Higher seden-

tary time is associated with IL-6 (an inflammatory cytokine) in men and women with type 2 diabetes, and reducing
sedentary time is associated with improved levels of CRP in
women.[10]

- **Toxins in the environment:** Chemicals in our environment can interfere with the immune system, paving the
  way for chronic inflammation. Studies have shown that
  exposure to pollution can cause adverse effects on health
  through increased oxidative stress, as well as changes in the
  inflammatory response and immune regulation.[11]

- **Gut dysbiosis and leaky gut:** When our gut health is out
  of whack, it's bad news for inflammation in all areas of our
  body. Research has shown that when the intestinal barrier
  gets damaged, it allows undigested food to leak into the
  bloodstream, triggering systemic inflammatory processes.[12]

As you can see, the most common triggers of chronic inflammation are all things that are somewhat within your control. And
it's no coincidence that the Immune Restoration Plan you're
going to follow is designed around the factors above.

GOT INFECTIONS?

The factors discussed above are very much under your control
and are lifestyle-related. But other causes of chronic inflammation are a little more mysterious and under the radar. In fact, one
of the most important root causes of immune imbalance and
chronic inflammation is the effect of an old, chronic, or hidden
infection that you may not even be aware of. The scientific literature has identified many viral and bacterial infections as triggers
for the development of diseases. Let's take one of the biggest

killers in the United States—heart attacks. There are plenty of lifestyle factors that contribute to heart disease (sugar, stress, smoking), but what about silent infections? In fact, patients with elevated antibodies to herpes virus (HSV-1) and the bacterium *Chlamydia pneumonia* have a higher risk of coronary heart disease. Other infections related to heart disease are *Porphyromonas gingivalis,* from periodontal disease, *Helicobacter pylori,* found in peptic ulcer disease, influenza A virus, hepatitis C virus, and cytomegalovirus (CMV).[13] [14] Interesting, isn't it?

Many autoimmune diseases are also linked to a previous or chronic infection.[15] This is due to several underlying mechanisms, including molecular mimicry, bystander activation, and viral persistence. In a nutshell, "molecular mimicry" means that part of the virus or bacteria may share some resemblance to human cells, so our immune system can get confused and attack our tissues when attacking the infection. This occurs in rheumatic heart disease and reactive arthritis in children stemming from an infection of strep throat, which can trigger antibodies directed against the heart muscle and joints.[16] Molecular mimicry is known to be triggered by many viruses, including hepatitis B and Epstein-Barr virus (EBV). In fact, recent studies found much higher rates of EBV in patients with systemic lupus.[17] "Bystander activation" refers to the activation of certain T cells that are hanging out in the area near a viral infection. Although these "bystanders" are not specific to the virus, they get triggered into action by the release of cytokines nearby. Sort of like immune peer pressure.

Lastly, "persistence" of viral and bacterial infections can lead to chronic immune activation because if the infection is not cleared, the immune system will stay on high alert. This is one of the ways in which nonresolving or undiagnosed Lyme disease can trigger autoimmune diseases such as rheumatoid arthritis.[18] [19] More recently, evidence is emerging for an autoimmune phenomenon occurring in some people infected with the SARS-CoV-2 virus, responsible for COVID-19.[20] In children with COVID-19, mysterious symptoms similar to that of the autoimmune disorder called Kawasaki disease started to show up, referred to as pediatric multisystem inflammatory syndrome.[21] In addition, other autoimmune diseases such as immune thrombocytopenia, thyroiditis, and Guillain-Barré syndrome are becoming more frequent in post–COVID-19 cases.[22] A recent yet-unpublished study has given even more credence to the theory that this virus is stimulating an autoimmune response in certain patients. One hundred and fifty-four post-COVID patients were found to have significant increases in autoantibodies against proteins found in their own cytokines and immune cells.[23] And although it's unclear whether this explains some of the symptoms seen in the COVID-19 "long haulers," it does indicate that this virus, along with others, can derail the immune system even after it's gone.[24]

AUTOPHAGY: OUR SECRET CELLULAR CLEANUP WEAPON

Earlier, we talked about how the inflammatory response can leave a mess behind. And when that mess becomes too much, chronic and unproductive inflammation ensues. Luckily, we have an incredible ongoing natural mechanism that is used to clean up damaged cells before they elicit an inflammatory response. This amazing process is called autophagy, otherwise known as "self-eating,"[25] and its main function is cellular recycling. Just like organizing your office by getting rid of redundant paper and junk can help you work more efficiently, or Marie Kondo–ing your closet to create a minimalist capsule wardrobe can speed up your morning routine, your cells can take out their trash and become healthier and more streamlined too. Autophagy is different from the garbage collecting that macrophages perform, because macrophages are called in response to an infection, dead cells, or toxic waste. Autophagy, on the other hand, happens in healthy cells and is akin to regular cellular maintenance. It helps maintain a tidy environment in our cells that prevents chronic inflammation from occurring in the first place. In autophagy, your cell is getting a tune-up so that it will live longer and not be tagged for destruction. Just like regular tune-ups for your car will keep it rolling for many years, autophagy is a way to prevent or hold off cell death.

In autophagy, old damaged proteins and cell parts are collected by something called a lysosome, which is like a small organ inside your cells, and dumped into a recycling bin of sorts. Here, the old damaged components are burned up and recycled for energy or transformed into brand-new cellular parts. Voilà! Autophagy also helps cells dump intracellular pathogens like viruses, parasites, and bacteria.[26] Research has also shown that autophagy helps prevent many chronic diseases like Alzheimer's disease, autoimmune disease, and cancer, and is key to longevity.[27] [28] [29] [30]

Focusing on increasing autophagy is a big part of the Immune Restoration Plan because it helps take a load off our immune system and reduces nonproductive inflammation. One of the simplest and cheapest ways to ramp up your autophagy game is to try out intermittent fasting. If you've ever wondered why the wellness world is so obsessed with fasting, autophagy is the answer.[31] Basically, when we restrict calories or spend extended periods of time without food, our glucose stores become scarce and our bodies need to find other sources of energy. This kick-starts the autophagy process. The end result is healthier cells, enhanced immune tolerance and activity, and less chronic disease.[32]

TAKING DOWN FREE RADICALS

When immune cells get called in to kill microbes, they use some pretty nasty chemicals to do the killing. This can result in the release of noxious substances called free radicals. These reactive substances are normal, but they need to be squelched or else they'll bounce around destroying your cells and DNA. Too many free radicals floating about causes oxidative stress, which is sort of akin to your cells rusting over time. There are other common sources of free radicals, such as ultraviolet radiation from sunshine and toxins that you eat, drink, and breathe. You even make free radicals as a by-product when your cells make energy, so it's something we all deal with daily. Nevertheless, we have a solution. The key to neutralizing free radicals before they do too much harm is antioxidants. We're going to take a deep look at antioxidants later when we talk more about nutrition, but just know that these wonderful substances, like vitamin C, vitamin A, and vitamin E, neutralize our free radicals and pack a huge anti-inflammatory and proautophagy punch. If we don't have a good supply of these on hand from our diet, inflammation and cell damage just keep marching along. Antioxidants don't just come from food. In fact, melatonin, which you probably already know as the "sleep hormone," is actually an antioxidant. And a strong one, too! There's an entire chapter about sleep coming up, where we will delve deeper into the major influence that sleep has on our immune balance.

You may be wondering: Can't I just take an antioxidant or melatonin supplement and achieve the same results? We have a saying in functional medicine. "You can't supplement your way out of bad health." It's a normal occurrence for people to show up in my office with shopping bags full of vitamins and nutritional powders, frustrated that they "didn't work" for whatever ailment they have. Supplements can help, but only if you've done the work of removing sources of pointless inflammation by changing your sleep patterns, reducing your stress, avoiding sugar and processed foods, removing toxins, and adding in antioxidant-rich foods such as brightly colored fruits and vegetables. Just as a prescription drug from your doctor is not going to take away your disease, one vitamin or twenty won't transform your health on their own.

INFLAMMATION AND THE FOUR IMMUNOTYPES

We've spent these first chapters learning about the immune dysfunction crisis, the chronic disease crisis, and the underlying mechanisms (ahem, inflammation) at play. We've learned about the importance of productive inflammation, the dangers of nonproductive inflammation, and how lifestyle factors can influence our ability to mount a healthy inflammatory response. As you may already have guessed by how much of this book I've spent talking about inflammation, inflammation plays a role in all four Immunotypes. For example:

- If you're one of the millions of Americans who are walking around with diabetes, Alzheimer's disease, heart disease, or another inflammation-based disease thanks to your **Smol-**

dering Immunotype, the root cause of your issues *is too much inflammation.*

- If you're one of the 14 to 23 million people estimated to have an autoimmune disease, thanks to your **Misguided Immunotype**, the root cause of your problem *is inflammation that is being redirected against your own cells and organs.*
- If you're one of the 50 million Americans who experience various types of allergies each year, thanks to your **Hyperactive Immunotype**, the root cause of your problem *is inflammation that is triggered too easily by harmless substances that are normal parts of our environment.*
- If you're one of the millions of Americans who have a hard time getting through winter without multiple colds or the flu or bronchitis, thanks to your **Weak Immunotype**, the core issue *is an inflammatory response that is not reacting quickly and efficiently enough to properly do its job.*

Inflammation is really at the root of it all—it's the source of the problem and how we're going to fix it, too. Now that you know this, it'll come as no surprise that rebalancing the inflammatory response is a huge part of the Immune Restoration Plan. But before we jump into that section of the book, it's time to get specific about your personal immune imbalances. Finally! The moment I know you've all been waiting for. It's time to identify your Immunotype.

CHAPTER 4

The Four Immunotypes Quiz

W e've covered a lot of ground. In fact, you now probably know more about inflammation and how your immune system works than 99 percent of the population. You also understand that crafting a well-oiled immune response is not simply about boosting your immunity. In fact, depending on what state you're in right now, that may be the exact opposite of what you want to do! You see, your immune system is multidimensional; it doesn't just go up and down. It goes backward, forward, sideways, and upside down. So sit quietly, close your eyes, and repeat this mantra: *balance*. That is the crux of what we're after. That said, in order to attain immune balance, you have to know where you're starting from. This is why I've developed the four Immunotypes, to help you understand where you are so you can get where you want to go. These four main types of immune dysfunction—Smoldering, Misguided, Hyperactive, and Weak—encompass the main imbalances of the immune system that are most frequently making us sick today. These immunotypes are not genetic or fixed for life. You have the power to transform your health and get back into balance with simple interventions that anyone can do. The key is to figure out where you're starting from.

Many of you may be wondering how, without coming into my office or having advanced lab tests performed, you're going to figure out which immunotype you are. Lucky for you, I've developed the Four Immunotypes Quiz, which you'll use to identify your dominant Immunotype. By looking at characteristics and symptoms you have and the types of diseases and illnesses that ail you, you can get a clear sense of which Immunotype you fall into — no expensive tests or doctors' appointments required. Once you take the quiz and tally your results, you can read the information corresponding to your Immunotype to get an idea of what steps you'll want to take next.

THE FOUR IMMUNOTYPES QUIZ

To use this quiz correctly, take each of the four parts and answer every question as honestly as possible. You may find that you fall into more than one Immunotype, and that's normal! Many of us have more than one imbalance in our immune system, and oftentimes these imbalances play off one another in a sort of snowball effect. If this is you, I recommend paying attention to your primary Immunotype (the one where you score the highest) and using the tools and recommendations in the second half of this book to work on balancing that primary type. Then, when you've completed your first round of the Immune Restoration Plan for your Immunotype, you should retake the quiz to see if any of your scores have shifted. You'll find that as you achieve more balance in one of your Immunotypes, the others start to find balance as well. Why is this? Well, because everything in the immune system is totally interconnected and doesn't work in a vacuum. For example: If Jane takes the quiz and finds that she scores really high in the Smoldering Immunotype section but also has some moderate scores in the Hyperactive Immunotype section, she should start with the plan for the Smoldering Immunotype first. After completing the Immune Restoration plan for the Smoldering Immunotype, she may find that her score has dropped significantly for both Immunotypes but that now her highest score is for the Hyperactive Immunotype. She now can pivot and focus on using the suggestions for the Hyperactive Immunotype.

If you find that you don't score high for any of the Immunotypes—congratulations! You likely have a very healthy immune system. That said, you should still use the recommendations in the second half of this book to decrease nonproductive inflammation and prevent silent imbalances that may be forming unbeknownst to you. As I said before, it can take years for an imbalance to finally reach the point where you experience noticeable symptoms from it.

So, without further ado, let's jump into the quiz. Grab a pencil and a sheet of paper to tally your score for each Immunotype. Give yourself a point for each statement you agree with in the list below.

SMOLDERING

☐ I have diabetes or high blood sugar.
☐ I have coronary artery disease, have had a heart attack, or have high blood pressure.

- ☐ I am obese or overweight (BMI greater than 30).
- ☐ I have high blood sugar.
- ☐ I exercise fewer than three times a week.
- ☐ I drink more than six servings of alcohol a week.
- ☐ I sleep fewer than six and a half hours a night regularly.
- ☐ I eat fast food or processed foods.
- ☐ I smoke tobacco in any form.
- ☐ I take three or more prescription medications.
- ☐ I have periodontal (gum) disease.
- ☐ I have arthritis or inflamed joints.
- ☐ I have acne rosacea or seborrheic dermatitis.
- ☐ I rarely get colds or flu.
- ☐ I have inflammatory bowel disease like Crohn's disease or ulcerative colitis.

MISGUIDED

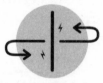

- ☐ I have been diagnosed with autoimmune disease.
- ☐ I have a family history of autoimmune disease (e.g., lupus, rheumatoid arthritis, or multiple sclerosis).
- ☐ I have joint pains that come and go or swollen joints.
- ☐ I have thyroid disease.
- ☐ Certain foods seem to make my symptoms flare up.
- ☐ Stress makes my symptoms flare.
- ☐ I have chronic muscle weakness or pain.

☐ I get tingling or numbness in my extremities or other neurologic symptoms.

☐ I have unexplained hair loss or thinning (not age-related).

☐ I have mysterious skin rashes that come and go.

☐ I have taken many antibiotics over my lifetime.

☐ I have dry mouth and/or dry eyes.

☐ I had childhood trauma or adverse events.

☐ I had mononucleosis as a child.

HYPERACTIVE

☐ I have seasonal or year-round allergies.

☐ I have food allergies or sensitivities.

☐ I have asthma or chronic cough.

☐ I have a history of ear infections.

☐ I have a history of sinusitis.

☐ I have physical reactions to strong scents or odors.

☐ I have eczema or other itchy rashes.

☐ I break out in hives or swelling.

☐ I have allergic reactions to medications.

☐ I am sensitive to mold.

☐ Personal care products like soap, lotion, or fragrance make me break out.

☐ I have a tendency to get yeast infections.

☐ I have a lot of postnasal drip or I clear my throat frequently.

☐ I've had bronchitis or pneumonia.

☐ I sneeze frequently.

WEAK

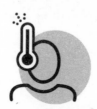

☐ I have a congenital or acquired immune deficiency (HIV).

☐ I have taken long-term (more than fourteen days) or fre-
    quent (more than twice a year) corticosteroids (predni-
    sone/cortisone).

☐ I take immunosuppressive medications (such as
    chemotherapy).

☐ I get frequent colds or upper-respiratory infections.

☐ I have had pneumonia more than once.

☐ I get frequent urinary tract infections.

☐ I have had shingles before the age of sixty or more than once.

☐ I get frequent outbreaks of herpes, including cold sores.

☐ I have chronic fatigue.

☐ It's common for me to get diarrhea or food poisoning
    when I travel.

☐ I often feel run-down.

☐ I have to sleep a lot or else I get sick.

☐ I get sick after a period of stress.

☐ My colds last for weeks.

Scoring: Tally up the number of statements you checked off for
each Immunotype. The type with the highest number is your

primary Immunotype, but you may score high in other Immuno-types as well. As I said, you may have characteristics of several. Focus on your dominant type in the following sections, which go into real-life examples of what it's like to have each Immunotype.

THE SMOLDERING IMMUNOTYPE

Greg was a fifty-five-year-old executive for a petrochemical company who came to my office after his primary care doctor told him he needed yet another medication to deal with his high blood pressure. He was also warned that he was "prediabetic" and might need medication for that soon too. Greg had always put his career first in his life, often working ten- to twelve-hour days, and had climbed the company ladder quickly into an influential position. He described himself as an adrenaline junkie, always up for a challenge, and loved closing a deal more than anything. He traveled extensively, often to China and South America, entertaining clients and eating out on expense accounts. Recently the jet lag had been getting harder for him to bounce back from, and he often found himself waking up at odd hours and usually getting no more than six hours of sleep a night.

He had done CrossFit workouts for a few years and liked it, but lately he had become quite sedentary due to his schedule. Nowadays he rarely found the time to get to the gym, and frankly, he didn't feel up to it anymore. He was also starting to forget people's names and didn't feel his thinking was as sharp as it used to be. His father had Alzheimer's disease, so this really worried him. To buoy his energy after a less-than-restful sleep, he started his day with "high-octane" Bulletproof coffee. He usually skipped breakfast or grabbed a granola bar, and picked up takeout for lunch, often getting more coffee and sometimes something sweet for an energy boost in the afternoon. When he wasn't doing client dinners, he sometimes made it home to eat dinner with his family, but this was often after 7 p.m. After a tough day it was common for him to have a whiskey or two glasses of red wine to relax. He loved his job but said the stress was getting to him. He was arguing more with his wife and his teenage son, and he felt like he was getting more impatient in general.

Over the past four years he had developed aches and pains in his knees, hands, and feet, for which he would pop a Tylenol or Advil. He had developed a skin condition called rosacea on his face, which his doctor attributed to his Irish heritage, and struggled with patches of psoriasis on his elbows. He often had heartburn and had been taking Prilosec "for years" on and off. At an executive physical two years earlier, his blood pressure had been 148/90, his triglycerides were 250, and his total cholesterol was 240. He was also borderline obese, having gained more than thirty pounds in two years. He had started on a diuretic and a beta-blocker for his blood pressure and a statin drug for his cholesterol. The diuretic made him urinate in the middle of the night, interrupting his sleep, and he also noticed erectile dysfunction more frequently. At his last medical visit, his fasting blood sugar had been 105 (normal is less than 80). Despite all of this, Greg said he hardly ever got sick from colds and, to his recollection, hadn't ever had the flu. He always thought of himself as tough and resilient.

I could see that Greg's habits and lifestyle were driving a lot of inflammation in his body and setting multiple diseases in motion. I ran an in-depth set of laboratory tests to get a more complete picture. Since he was on a statin, his total cholesterol was 160, but his high-density lipoproteins (HDL) were only 48. HDL, which is often called the "good" cholesterol, is protective because it helps move cholesterol out of the body. You can drive up HDL levels with regular aerobic exercise. Greg also had high amounts of oxidized LDL, which is "damaged" cholesterol that leads to inflammation of the blood vessels. His C-reactive protein level was 12; it ideally should be less than 1. Elevations in C-reactive protein are one of the best indicators we have to assess systemic inflammation. Another blood marker called homocysteine was 22, which is about four times normal and is not only a big risk factor for cardiac disease but is often reversible with simple B vitamin supplementation.

Greg's insulin was also way out of range at 32. I call insulin the canary in the coal mine for diabetes. Doctors rarely check it, instead relying on fasting blood glucose and hemoglobin A1c for diagnosing diabetes. But insulin levels sometimes start to become chronically elevated years before diabetes is diagnosed. High levels indicate insulin resistance, as the pancreas tries desperately to keep serum blood sugar low. High insulin also prevents weight loss because it tells the body to stop burning fat. Excess blood sugar "glycates," or coats, red blood cells and damages blood vessels, triggering the inflammation response of the immune system. Lastly, I tested sex and adrenal hormone levels, as I do for all my clients. Greg had only moderately elevated cortisol, which is our main stress hormone, but his circadian pattern of cortisol was completely disordered. (We'll talk more about why this is so important in Chapter 6.) His morning cortisol was too low, but it would shoot up in late morning, tank in the afternoon, and then be elevated again around bedtime. Cortisol is a major mediator of inflammation in the body. As we'll learn later, it can be both pro- and anti-inflammation. However, with all the imbalances in Greg's labs and his symptoms, he was clearly a Smoldering immunotype.

If some (or all!) of Greg's story feels familiar to you and you scored more than five points on the Smoldering Immunotype part of the quiz, the root cause of your issues is too much inflammation throwing the entire body out of whack. Those with a Smoldering Immunotype don't always have a diagnosable disease, nor are they sick enough that they have to stay home from work or cancel their day, but they typically have a lot of little things going wrong at the same time. For example, a little bit of insomnia, aches and pains, brain fog, some chronic stress, occasional sexual dysfunction, and labs that are in the "worrisome" category but not necessarily in the "needs medication" category.

If you have a Smoldering Immunotype, pay attention to all of the Smoldering-specific advice in the second half of the book. The good news about this Immunotype is that with a few key lifestyle changes, you can reverse this negative cycle of inflammation, and your symptoms should improve rapidly! Remember that out-of-control inflammation is at the core of so many diseases that we suffer from today, like heart disease, metabolic syndrome and obesity, diabetes, autoimmune diseases, and Alzheimer's, to name a few. Also, once your inflammation is under control, your immune system can pay attention to the really important things, like effectively killing dangerous microbes and helping you live a long, healthy life.

THE MISGUIDED IMMUNOTYPE

Rachel was a young attorney who was diagnosed with rheumatoid arthritis at twenty-six, about a year after starting her job at a law firm. She was under a lot of stress at the time, as she had just broken up with her long-term boyfriend, and she was a self-identified perfectionist who worked sometimes as late as 10 p.m. at the office and took work home on the weekends. Initially, she just took Advil daily for the pain and stiffness in her hands, which she attributed to typing all day and going to her 6 a.m. kickboxing classes. After she started to see swelling in her knuckles and pain in her feet, she went to her doctor, who ordered hand X-rays and lab tests. Her X-rays were consistent with early rheumatoid changes, so her doctor ordered an anti–cyclic citrullinated peptide (anti-CCP) antibodies test, which tests for active rheumatoid arthritis, and started her on prednisone and then methotrexate. After minimal changes, her doctor recommended an immune-modulating drug called Humira. Rachel had heard about reversing autoimmune issues with more "natural measures," so she came to me.

As we dug into her backstory, I found that she'd had a pretty uneventful childhood, except that she had recurrent strep throat infections and remembered going to the doctor a lot for antibiotics. She was on the cross-country team and said she didn't have a healthy relationship with food. She dropped so much weight when she was sixteen years old that she didn't get her period for nine months. She also had acne as a teen and was teased for her pimples. After trying many creams and oral minocycline (an antibiotic), she went on Accutane for a year and birth control pills, which cleared her skin completely. After college, she traveled in Thailand and Vietnam for several weeks and got very sick with diarrhea and fever, which resolved without treatment. After starting law school, she noticed increasing gas and bloating after meals and more frequent bouts of loose stool. Her doctor diagnosed her with irritable bowel syndrome and she started on Linzess (an antispasmodic) for her symptoms. After reading information online, Rachel cut out gluten and dairy and felt a little better but would still vacillate between running to the bathroom and getting really constipated when stressed.

When she came to the office, Rachel said she was tired all the time despite how much she slept and was feeling anxious and unmotivated. She wondered whether law was really the best career for her and sometimes felt foggy and couldn't concentrate at work. In addition, she had frequent yeast infections and occasional urinary tract infections. She hated taking antibiotics but felt like she had to several times a year.

Given her GI symptoms, I ordered a microbiome stool test, which showed high levels of a bacterium called *Klebsiella pneumoniae,* a known autoimmune instigator.[1] In addition, she had low levels of several protective gut bacteria such as *Bifidobacterium* and *Lactobacillus* and high levels of *Candida albicans*—a type of yeast— all indicating a microbiome imbalance. Food sensitivity testing revealed antibodies to soy, gluten, and cow's milk. Despite her having normal thyroid hormone levels, we also discovered high antibodies to her thyroid gland, indicating that she was moving toward developing an autoimmune condition of the thyroid called Hashimoto's thyroiditis. Rachel was a perfect example of a Misguided Immunotype.

If you've been diagnosed with an autoimmune disease, it's a safe bet that like Rachel, you have a Misguided Immunotype. As you can see, a Misguided Immunotype doesn't just pop up overnight; it's the result of many factors, but especially stress and gut microbiome imbalances, infections, and toxins. If you have a Misguided Immunotype and currently struggle with an autoimmune condition, your doctor may have told you that medication is your only answer—and that you're destined to experience pain, discomfort, and other symptoms for the rest of your life. I'm here to tell you that medication is not the *only* thing that can help you. I've seen dozens of patients with a Misguided Immunotype improve their life by making diet and lifestyle changes. Some of them have even gone into remission from their autoimmune condition or eliminated the need for medications.

If Rachel's health history sounds like your own, whether you have a diagnosed autoimmune disease, autoimmune disease runs in your family, or you suspect you might be developing one, pay close attention to the chapter on gut health (Chapter 7). More than 70 percent of your immune system lives in your gut, and you need your microbes to be working with you—not against you—if you want to heal from a Misguided Immunotype!

THE HYPERACTIVE IMMUNOTYPE

Kelly was a thirty-two-year-old artist who noticed some shortness of breath when she was out running one spring day. An avid runner, she didn't normally suffer from any breathing issues but knew that as a child she'd had mild asthma that she had "grown out of." She was referred to a pulmonologist, who diagnosed her as having exercise-induced asthma, and was prescribed an albuterol inhaler to use before she ran. She felt this helped, but now she was having some coughing and wheezing when she was in her ceramics studio. She also started getting a postnasal drip and a stuffy nose, which seemed to worsen when she was working. As far back as she remembered, she'd had sneezing and itchy eyes in the spring and summer. She recalled that she had been on allergy shots for pollen and dust for a few years in her teens, but stopped when she went to college. She was taking the antihistamine Zyrtec on a daily basis. It helped a little but sometimes made her eyes feel dry. It didn't seem to be helping her current symptoms enough to make her feel at her best. As a child, she'd had eczema behind her knees and in the creases of her elbows. She didn't have that now, but she often broke out in hives "randomly" and always when she was around cats. She tried to use hypoallergenic beauty products because her skin was sensitive and would break out if she used perfumed lotions, soaps, or laundry detergent.

Over the past several years, she'd started getting sinus

infections at least twice a year, usually when her allergies were the worst. They would often take weeks to clear and require a round of steroids and antibiotics to clear them up. They were so bad she was considering sinus surgery, as recommended by her ENT (ear, nose, and throat) doctor. And although she didn't know of any food allergies in her past, Kelly had noticed in recent years that eating eggs made her nauseous and certain nuts would make her mouth and throat itch a little, so she just avoided them.

Lab testing revealed a total IgE antibody level of 850, which was markedly elevated. As I discussed in Chapter 2, IgE is the antibody that instigates the release of histamine, causing all sorts of allergic symptoms like sneezing, stuffiness, and even anaphylaxis. Kelly also had allergy blood tests showing positive reactions to tree and ragweed pollen, cat dander, and dust mites.

If some of Kelly's story resonates with you and you scored high on the Hyperactive Immunotype part of the quiz, you likely have a Th2 polarization. In the Immune Restoration Plan, you'll focus on the recommendations to bolster a Th1 response, as well as using interventions designed to dampen the biochemistry of allergies.

THE WEAK IMMUNOTYPE

When Bill came to see me, he was on his fourth antibiotic of the year and it was only March. He had had a sinus infection that didn't seem to want to budge, as well as two bouts of bronchitis. He was really worried that at the age of thirty-five, he had a weak immune system, and he wanted to see what he could do to stop getting sick so much. He thought the uptick in illness might be because he had two small children who often brought viruses home from school and the fact that in the past year, he had been under a lot of financial stress. He had left his job to start his own business, and it was struggling. He worked long hours and often stayed up past midnight on his laptop to get work done. He woke up tired and often felt the need to nap in the afternoons. He said he was a little bit of a germaphobe because he seemed to get sick pretty easily, so he used a lot of hand sanitizer and avoided crowds when he could. He described himself as a worrier and had always been anxious, but he took an SSRI (Serotonin re-uptake inhibitor medication) to help with that. In the past he had trained for several marathons, which helped with his moods, but now he didn't have the time or energy to do so.

Growing up, he said, he got colds fairly easily and had "walking pneumonia" as a teenager. His parents told him that he was born prematurely and was given some medication for his "weak" lungs. He also contracted mononucleosis in his freshman year of college and missed about a month of school. He said he had always had a sensitive stomach, but his bowels seemed to be more irregular lately, with occasional diarrhea. He suspected that certain foods he was eating were causing bloating, but he couldn't pinpoint which ones. He had experienced food poisoning several times in the past, so he was careful to avoid buffet restaurants and sushi, and he washed his produce carefully. He had also contracted giardia (an intestinal parasite) while camping with friends in Northern California several years before.

His laboratory testing revealed relatively normal immunoglobulin levels, but despite having received a pneumonia vaccine in January, he did not have adequate antibody response to it. In addition, he tested positive for high levels of a specific form of antibody to the Epstein-Barr virus, which can indicate a reactivation and increased replication of the virus in the body. His stool testing revealed a low level of secretory IgA, which is the primary protective antibody in the intestinal tract. In addition, he had very low levels of certain protective bacteria, such as *Bifidobacte-rium* and *Lactobacillus*. His cortisol levels were somewhat flatlined. They started out moderate in the morning but went down and stayed that way throughout the day. In addition, his overnight urine levels of melatonin were extremely low. Clearly, Bill was having problems fighting off both viral and bacterial infections, and he had a poor response to vaccines. In addition, he was exhausted and sleep-deprived and had the depressed cortisol output often seen with ongoing chronic stress and immune suppression. He fell clearly into the Weak Immunotype category.

If you can relate to Bill's story and you scored highest in the Weak Immunotype category, you can relate to the feeling of "catching everything" that goes around. There's a good chance you're wary of germs, have a hard time recovering quickly from being sick, and often suffer from back-to-back illnesses, like strep throat and then a sinus infection and then bronchitis—all seemingly one after another. If you have a Weak Immunotype, you might feel like you're destined to be this way. But that's not true! By making some key changes to your routine and taking some targeted supplements to boost the immune system, you can help your immune system respond more efficiently to all sorts of invaders. Weak immunotypes usually need to strengthen the activity of both innate and adaptive immune responses. Pay attention to any advice in the second half of the book that is specifically designed to "boost" the immune system—you're in the group that can benefit from this!

Don't worry if the cases I provided don't fit you *exactly;* that's okay. We're all individuals and genetically different from one another, and you don't have to have every single symptom in common with Greg or Rachel or Kelly or Bill. Now that you've read real-life examples of how all four Immunotypes can occur, it's time to talk about *how* we're going to shift you out of imbalance and back into immune harmony. We already know that there are four distinct immune patterns and that those patterns have everything to do with T cell polarization. Well, one of the major targets of the Immune Restoration Plan is reversing and rebalancing this polarization to restore healthy immune function, so let's dive deeper into this important part of the puzzle.

T CELL POLARIZATION AND THE FOUR IMMUNOTYPES

So far in this book we've talked a lot about how your immune system works and what can go wrong. Back in Chapter 2, I introduced the concept of "T cell polarization," one of the most important underlying mechanisms that leads to the four Immunotypes. Every day your immune system reacts as it deals with different threats like viruses, bacteria, parasites, irritants, toxins, foods, stress, sleep deprivation, etc. Depending on how chronic these triggers are and how your immune system responds, your immune system can develop tendencies that can start to throw it out of balance. These tendencies are called T cell polarization or dominance, and they allow you to mount precise immune responses against whatever enemy is present. But when T cell polarization gets imbalanced in one direction, you can end up stuck in one continuous loop. These continuous T cell polarization loops are at the heart of the Immunotypes and what we'll be targeting with the Immune Restoration Plan.

Let's talk in even more detail about what's going on here: Your helper T cells are the head honchos of your adaptive immune response, because they essentially direct everything. They secrete cytokines, tell the killer T cells what to do, and direct your B cells to make antibodies against germs. Remember, your innate initial immune response is pretty much fixed (as soon as something foreign enters your body, an army of cells like macrophages, neutrophils, and other cells will rush to the scene, check out the problem, and engulf and kill invaders if necessary), but your adaptive immune response tailors itself to the specific threat (T cells and B cells pump out cytokines, directly kill microbes, make memory clones of themselves to fight infections later, and create antibodies that recognize future infections). Because the cells of our innate immune system, such as the dendritic cells, are the ones on the front line, they will snip off and deliver a piece of whatever invader is causing the problem over to our lymph nodes, and a custom helper T cell is made just for the job. It's like your dendritic cells arrive and say "Hey! We've got an adenovirus making trouble in the sinuses, or a giardia parasite that made its way into the intestines from that river water! Who's up for the job?"

We learned in Chapter 2 about four main helper T cell subtypes—Th1, Th2, TH17, and regulatory T cells. Let's go into more depth on what each one means and how it influences your Immunotype.

- **TH1:** Th1 cells are created in response to bacteria and viruses that get inside and invade our cells. Once a naïve T cell is polarized into its Th1 form, it produces gobs of inflammatory cytokines, which help recruit cytotoxic T cells and NK cells. We make a lot of Th1 cells when we're trying to kill viruses and bacteria that have invaded our cells. Although we want to be able to make lots of Th1 cells for a vigorous immune response, we also don't want it to get out of control. When people get stuck in a Th1 dominance, they can become overly inflamed. This can lead to problems ranging from arthritis and diabetes to heart disease, and a number of autoimmune diseases. On the other hand, people who have a strong Th1 dominance tend to not get a lot of respiratory illnesses or have many allergies. Such people may have a Smoldering or Misguided Immunotype or both. People with a Weak Immunotype often benefit from having more Th1 cells, as they need help clearing out infections; and those with a Hyperactive Immunotype may also need more Th1 activity to balance themselves out.

- **TH2:** Th2 cells are activated when we're dealing with invading parasites, as well as bacteria that replicate in cavities and on surfaces of the body. Think sinus and bladder infections. Toxins like heavy metals also trigger this type of immune response. Th2 cells make cytokines that recruit immune cells into the area, and stimulate B cells to produce IgE, the allergic antibody. This is done to kill and clear out the offending pathogen. Because of this, people who have a Th2 dominance may tend to have asthma, eczema, food allergies, sinusitis, and other allergic diseases. IgE antibodies cause the release of histamine and lead to allergic symptoms like hives, runny nose, swelling, nasal congestion, and excess mucus. Really this is just an immune response gone awry. Th2-dominant people tend to fall into the Hyperactive Immunotype. Some can also develop autoimmune issues down the line, when they cannot clear infections or other triggers.

- **TH17:** Th17 cells were discovered only a short time ago by researchers looking at the underlying cause of autoimmune disease. Originally, scientists thought that Th1 cells were the big drivers in autoimmune disease, until they found that Th17 cells were the true culprits.[2] Th17 cells secrete highly inflammatory cytokines, which are critical in fighting certain bacteria, yeast, and other fungal infections; but they also promote autoimmune activity and have been correlated with inflammatory bowel disease, Sjögren's syndrome, multiple sclerosis, lupus, and rheumatoid arthritis.[3] [4] [5] Most Misguided Immunotypes will have excessive Th17 polarization.

- **Regulatory T cells:** T-reg cells are the fourth and final population of helper T cells. These cells are the off switch to our immune response, and if we didn't have them we'd be in big trouble. Specifically, they encourage our immune system to ignore or "tolerate" the body's own tissues; this is crucial in preventing autoimmune disease and allergies.[6] T-reg cells can often be hijacked by cancer cells, allowing cancer to spread under the radar of the immune system. These guys are the yin to our yang. Like mediators, they calm down a lot of other inflammatory responses and can balance out-of-control immune reactions. We definitely want to have a lot of regulatory T cells to keep the peace, but not so much that we can't mount a strong immune response and kill dangerous threats. Increasing the amount of T-reg cells in the Smoldering, Misguided, and Hyperactive Immunotypes can help balance these types. We're going to talk about interventions to do just that.

So let's recap. As we move into the Immune Restoration Plan section of this book, remember that in order to create the best immune system, we're going to be working on a cellular level. This is how we're going to do that:

1. First and foremost, you'll get rid of unnecessary inflammation that is distracting your immune system from the important stuff.

2. You'll nourish and support your innate immune cells so they can do their job quickly and efficiently.

3. You'll rebalance any out-of-whack T cell polarization that may be pushing you toward certain symptoms and diseases. And while there isn't a perfect correlation between these four types of helper T cells and the four Immunotypes, you can't optimize your health without focusing on this area.

On a positive note, T cell polarization is largely driven by outside influences, so it's not set in stone. For example, it's affected by chemicals and toxins in our environment, our diet, stress, and chronic infections. In a perfect immune system—one that is not Smoldering, Misguided, Hyperactive, or Weak—our innate and adaptive teams are perfectly coordinated, swiftly and specifically protecting us from harm. That's what we're aiming for with the Immune Restoration Plan.

HEADING INTO THE IMMUNE RESTORATION PLAN

Now that you've familiarized yourself with the inner workings of your own immune system army, learned all about chronic inflammation and the way it contributes to the four Immunotypes, and identified your own Immunotype, it's time to investigate the factors that affect the health of your immune system—sleep, stress, gut health, toxins in your environment, and your diet. Until now we've been taking a big-picture approach to the immune system, but now we're about to get über-practical. In the upcoming pages, I'll connect those five major lifestyle factors to the health of your immune system and give you real, practical advice on how to

improve your lifestyle so that it starts helping your immune system instead of hurting it. We'll be delving into the major lifestyle
factors that affect immune health. And I just want to warn you,
there's a lot to cover! Don't feel like you need to remember everything or do it all. In fact, to prevent information overload, I created an "At a Glance" chapter later on in the book, which outlines
the best recommendations for each Immunotype.

Are you ready? Let's get started.

Part II

THE IMMUNE RESTORATION PLAN

CHAPTER 5

Sleep: Power Down Your Body, Power Up Your Immune System

About ten years ago I was training for an Ironman triathlon, commuting and working full-time as an allergist, completing an integrative medicine fellowship, and still trying to have a social life. It was typical for me to wake at 5 a.m. to get to the pool or to meet my training partners for a 5:20 a.m. bike ride. After a full day I would sit in front of my computer until late in the evening, often hitting the pillow after 11 p.m. I routinely clocked between six and six and a half hours of sleep a night because I had so much to fit in and I thought I could "cheat the system." Little did I know, I was the one being duped.

At the time, I didn't understand that sleep was so crucial to my health. I didn't realize that without deep sleep, my muscles weren't clearing out lactic acids from all the intense endurance exercise, and my cell repair and muscle recovery were impaired, setting me up for injury. I also didn't grasp that less REM sleep impaired my memory, not only decreasing my capacity to learn and remember but also aging my brain faster. Without adequate sleep, my stress hormones were getting dysregulated, affecting my weight, mood, and gut health. Now, years later, I've become a sleep evangelist. Why? Because I know that restful sleep is the cornerstone not just of a healthy immune system but of a healthy body in general.

Getting eight hours of sleep every night seems like an obvious and simple task at first glance, doesn't it? But so many of us try to get around it, whether we're too busy with work, we prioritize our social lives, or we engage in habits that keep us up at night staring at the ceiling. Getting great sleep is low-hanging fruit when it comes to improving our health, and yet, somehow, so many of us struggle with it. I see patients all the time who go to the gym every day, eat an incredibly healthy diet, cook all their meals at home, and have made sacrifices like eliminating alcohol or sugar from their lives but *still* can't manage to get great sleep. In fact, a whopping 50 million Americans suffer from some type of sleep disorder (for the record, that's more people than live in New York and Texas combined), and one in three adults in the US gets less than the minimum recommended seven hours of sleep a night. This, sadly, is affecting our health in more ways than one. Why? Because sleep deprivation doesn't just make us feel tired the next day, it actually creates inflammation and oxidative stress and increases our risk for disease. The famous saying "I'll sleep when I'm dead" takes on a whole new meaning when you learn that sleep deprivation is linked to increased rates of hypertension, heart disease, obesity, diabetes, depression, and cancer. Since this is a book about the immune system, it should come as no surprise that sleep deprivation also damages your ability to fend off pathogens and contributes to autoimmune disease, allergies, and chronic inflammation. In other words, sleep deprivation directly contributes to the imbalances seen in all four Immunotypes. All of the complex components of your immune system army rely on adequate sleep and a healthy circadian rhythm to work effectively. So many of us are shortchanging our health and increasing our risk for disease every night by not mastering the art of a great night's sleep.

DEMYSTIFYING THE CIRCADIAN CLOCK

I know many of you will be reading the paragraph above, thinking: "Well, don't we all need a different amount of sleep?" Although we all have differing sleep "chronotypes"—that is, some of us are fervent night owls and some of us are annoying morning larks (including yours truly)—humans are designed to sleep at night and be awake during the day when there is natural light. This is because all of our bodily functions are driven by a circadian rhythm set by a central pacemaker of sorts that's hidden away in an area of the brain called the suprachiasmatic nucleus.[1] This central clock—you may also have heard it referred to as your "body clock" or "circadian clock"—runs on an approximately twenty-four-hour schedule based on the Earth's rotation around the sun. I say "approximately" because our bodies aren't like normal clocks that count the minutes; instead, it's our exposure to light that resets our body clocks perfectly like a Swiss watch each day. Every morning when you blink your eyes open, light waves flood your retinas and adjust the central clock in your brain to tell your brain and body that it's morning now. This signal also synchronizes all the "mini-clocks" in the tissues and cells of your body, which help regulate your hormones, digestion, and immune system.[2] (This is one of the reasons why flying across time zones or even springing forward from standard time to daylight saving time is so disruptive to our bodies.)

At the end of the day, as the sun is going down, your brain's pineal gland starts to ramp up your main regulator of sleep and wakefulness—the hormone melatonin. Melatonin is an antioxidant that prevents cell damage but also regulates certain proinflammatory cytokines, playing an immune-balancing role.[3] It's extremely low during the day, but as darkness falls, it climbs and sets into motion many important changes in the body that not only make us sleepy and relaxed but also affect our blood sugar, body temperature, and blood pressure. But here's the catch: Small amounts of light can prevent melatonin from appropriately surging in the evening. Even the light from an incandescent lightbulb on your bedside table can disrupt melatonin, sabotaging your ability to fall asleep.

Even worse than your bedside lamp is the effect of short-wavelength (blue) light on your melatonin production and sleep. In 1988, scientists discovered a specialized melanopsin cell in our retina that is exquisitely sensitive to short-wave blue light.[4] During the day, blue light is stimulating and helps us with attention and mood. But in the evening when we're exposed to this wavelength, the pineal gland shuts down production of melatonin quickly, knocking our circadian rhythm out of balance.[5] Unfortunately, blue light is emitted from all LED lights, like those coming from our watches, computers, tablets, smartphones, and TVs. Even as we try to fall asleep we're bathed in blue light from the indicator lights on humidifiers, chargers, baby monitors, alarm clocks, and air-conditioning units in our bedrooms. It's no wonder we can't sleep!

Ninety percent of Americans report using some sort of blue-light-emitting tech device before bedtime, and the more involved the activity—such as texting, working on a computer, or video gaming—the harder it is to fall asleep and the less refreshed you are in the morning.[6] Even passively reading a screen can be a problem. In 2014, a study at Harvard examined the effects of reading on an e-reader compared with reading a printed book. The group using the e-readers took longer to fall asleep and had reduced REM sleep (the dream phase when you store memory) compared to the people who read old-fashioned print books. Even after sleeping eight hours, the e-reading folks took longer to wake up and felt more tired.[7] I don't want to put all the blame for insomnia and poor sleep quality on blue light, as there are many other factors that get in the way of our getting quality shut-eye, but our personal daily light pollution plays a crucial role.

THE IMMUNE SYSTEM DURING SLEEP

You might be wondering why I'm spending all this time talking about the circadian rhythm and blue light. Well, despite being a quiet time for other parts of your body, sleep is a *very active time for your immune system*. This might seem strange at first, so let's dive into the different phases of sleep and what your body is doing during each.

Your sleep is divided into different phases, and your body performs different functions during each. When you first fall asleep at night, you enter non–rapid eye movement sleep, which is when your muscles begin to relax and your breathing slows. Then you enter deep sleep, when your body is in a highly activated immune state. At night, the naïve T cells in your lymph nodes are presented with new antigens that your innate immune cells have picked up during the day; your NK cells are busy killing viruses and trolling for cancer cells; and your B cells are pumping out antibodies. During deep sleep it's normal to have higher levels of proinflammatory cytokines like TNF-α, IL-1 and IL-6, which are triggered by melatonin and direct your immune cells to attack and kill anything that has found its way into your body during the day. One of the reasons that this proinflammatory atmosphere takes over during sleep is the absence of high amounts of the stress hormone cortisol. Cortisol is at its lowest during the night, so its strong anti-inflammatory effects don't interfere with all of this immune activity.[8]

All this inflammatory frenzy might be taking place at night when we're asleep because inflammation in all its forms is not that convenient to experience during the day.[9] Think about it: being achy, in pain, tired, and feverish isn't conducive to exercise, working, socializing, or doing much more than remaining in the fetal position on your sofa. Did you ever wonder why getting a fever is more common at night, or why you sleep so much when you're sick? That's thanks to all those nocturnal cytokines doing their job killing things. This cycle of immune activity and sleep is also a two-way street. When we get infected with a virus or bacteria, our immune response causes changes in our brain that actually make us sleepy. Experiments in which human volunteers were injected with low-level endotoxins from bacteria showed that non-REM (NREM) sleep increased.[10] Our body and brain really tell us to sleep when we're under attack by an infection, and they do that through these sleep-inducing cytokines.[11] In addition, during NREM sleep the thermoregulatory systems of our body are in a place where fever can readily occur to help fight off bacteria and viruses. Fever is stimulated by several proinflammatory cytokines, such as interferon gamma (IFN-γ) and TNF-α, and has been shown to improve outcomes. But here's the catch: You can only have a sleeping nighttime fever if you're in deep sleep. Why? Because a fever requires shivering, a bodily function that is blocked in REM sleep and can only happen in certain deep sleep phases of NREM sleep.[12]

All this nighttime immune activation requires a lot of energy. The body needs fuel to make new proteins, pump out fresh cells, and make heaps of antibodies. Luckily, while we sleep our basal metabolic rate is lower and our muscles aren't burning up as much glucose as when we're running around during the day. This allows our immune system to siphon off this surplus energy and get to work. This system really is amazing! It's like the body has thought of everything. Even the waste generated by all this nighttime inflammation—in the form of free radicals that damage cells and produce oxidative stress—is taken care of by none other than melatonin, which acts not only as the sleep hormone but also as a potent antioxidant and free-radical scavenger.[13]

SLEEP DEPRIVATION AND THE IMMUNE SYSTEM

At the same time that proper sleep allows for a controlled environment of immune activity and inflammation, long-term sleep deprivation deregulates this response and causes chronic inflammation and disease. Sleep loss is associated with a vast range of inflammatory disease states, including obesity.[14] This occurs because our hunger hormones are thrown off when we don't sleep. For example, the hormone ghrelin, which increases hunger signals to the brain, goes up when we're sleep-deprived. In addition, our satiety hormone, leptin, goes down, so we're hungry but feel less satisfied when we eat. Obesity is itself a chronic inflammatory condition, because adipose (fat) cells secrete their own entourage of proinflammatory chemicals called adipokines. In fact, obese individuals can have a threefold increase in tumor necrosis factor alpha (TNF-α), interleukin 6 (IL-6), and C-reactive protein (CRP), all further contributing to chronic disease and accelerated aging. Yikes. So you can think of sleep as a great way to lower inflammation and prevent weight gain. In fact, it's the cheapest and most pleasurable weight loss technique—make sure you sleep eight hours!

Another way in which sleep loss contributes to both obesity and another inflammatory disease, type 2 diabetes, is by wreaking havoc on your nighttime blood sugar levels. Several studies have shown that over time, as short-sleepers get older, the risk of type 2 diabetes and obesity increases. One study took eleven young men and restricted them to four hours of sleep a night for six nights. The study measured their glucose tolerance after the last day and compared these results to those taken after the same participants were allowed twelve hours in bed for six nights. The results were startling. After the sleep deprivation the men's glucose tolerance plummeted, while their stress hormones surged.[15] Frankly, even a less-severe sleep restriction will do this. Another study compared the glucose tolerance of healthy individuals who got less than six and a half hours per night to people who got between seven and a half and eight and a half hours per night. At first the glucose tolerance looked the same in the two groups, but the short-sleepers secreted an average of 50 percent more insulin just to keep their blood sugar balanced.[16] This is the kind of pattern that over time leads to insulin resistance and eventually diabetes, just from skimping on a few hours of sleep.

Chronically poor sleep stresses us out—it increases our stress hormone cortisol and sends our body into fight-or-flight mode. Cortisol should be at its lowest at night while we sleep and does not start to increase until around 2 a.m., peaking in the early-morning hours. However, if it's elevated in the middle of the night it tells our body we're in an emergency situation rather than relaxing and restoring from the previous day. Cortisol triggers the release of glucose from organs as if we need to fight or flee.[17] This is why our blood sugar can spike in the nighttime, increasing the risk for diabetes and other diseases over time.

So you can see by now that our immune system is very active at night under the reign of our main sleep hormone, melatonin, and that sleep deprivation throws a wrench into this balance, throwing off blood sugar and hormones and leading to development of diseases like diabetes and obesity. It's a vicious cycle, too, because as we get more inflamed, our immune system weakens. One of the things we learned from the COVID-19 pandemic is how much preexisting conditions drive diminishing immune response. People with diabetes, heart disease, hypertension, obesity, and other comorbid conditions have higher rates of hospitalization and death not just from COVID-19 but from most serious infections.[18] Simply put, an overinflamed body and an unhealthy immune system cannot successfully fight and recover from a powerful novel virus.[19]

I bet you can recall a time when you skipped out on sleep for a few days and ended up sick with a cold. That's because inadequate sleep can sabotage the immune system immediately. In fact, research has shown that even one night of sleep deprivation can reduce NK cell activity and cytokine levels that fight viral infections. In one study, two groups were given a hepatitis A vaccine in the morning, and then they either pulled an all-nighter or had a normal night's sleep. Four weeks later, the folks with the full night's sleep had a twofold higher antibody production than the sleep-deprived group.[20] Similar results were found when people with insomnia or chronic sleep loss received the flu shot.[21] If you're regularly getting fewer than seven hours of sleep a night, you're almost three times more likely to catch the common cold than if you sleep more than eight hours a night.[22] Even more concerning, studies show that cancer patients who sleep poorly have higher mortality rates, probably due to weaker cancer-patrolling NK cells.[23]

Clearly, there's an intricate connection between sleep and the immune system, as it relates to both chronic disease and our ability to fight off acute infections. But here's the good news: As soon as you start getting high-quality sleep, your immune system rebounds swiftly. For example, studies have shown that after just one night of recovery sleep, NK cell activity returns to normal levels.[24] In addition, one night of great sleep can lead to better blood sugar levels, lower stress hormones, and fewer cravings for unhealthy foods the next day. You'll also experience better concentration, a more positive mood, and higher energy levels. These immediate benefits are some of the most amazing things about sleep and why it's so important to optimizing health. We may think we have to work for months before we see improvements in our health. And that can be true when it comes to eating more healthily, exercising, or taking a new supplement or medication. But when it comes to sleep, improving your sleep *tonight* could lead to measurable improvements in your health and well-being as soon as tomorrow morning. Pretty cool, isn't it?

YOUR SLEEP TOOLKIT

Regardless of which Immunotype you fall into, you'll need to maximize your sleep to keep chronic disease and acute infections at bay. I've noticed that different people benefit from different sleep tools. Approach the following Sleep Toolkit from the perspective of which tips and tricks will help you as an individual based on your schedule and where you need to change your habits. These interventions are not type-specific to your Immunotype; instead, pay attention to the places where you have room for improvement. After all, you do spend about a third of your life in bed! You might be shocked by how much all these small things work together to improve your sleep. Are you ready? Let's get to work!

If you want to upgrade your sleep, there are three things you absolutely must do. They include making sleep a priority, creating a healthy sleep environment, and winding down before bed.

1. Reprioritize sleep in your life.

To reap the benefits of blissful sleep, the place to start is with your priority list. We need to stop thinking of sleep as something we can skimp on or sacrifice in order to accomplish other (more important) goals. Repeat after me: Sleep is not negotiable. The National Sleep Foundation recommends that adults get between seven and nine hours of sleep a night; routinely getting less than seven hours of sleep a night may increase your risk for many diseases.[25] Your specific need will vary based on your age and state of health. Also, the quality of your sleep and how much time you actually sleep while lying in bed all weigh into this equation. A good rule of thumb is to aim for eight to eight and a half hours to ensure that you get that minimum of seven hours. If you've convinced yourself that you don't have enough time to sleep, I challenge you to track how you spend your time for a full twenty-four hours. You might be shocked by how much time you spend surfing the web, watching TV, shopping online, and doing other things that aren't bringing much benefit to your life. Once you've gotten honest about how you're spending your time, think about how you can cut down on those nonessential activities and reappropriate time for sleep instead.

One effective way to cut down on mindless scrolling is to set daily time limits on the apps on your phone. Most phones have this function already built in. By setting alerts or limits on certain apps on your phone, not only will you be prevented from wasting time scrolling, but you'll also see how much time you're spending on these activities. In addition, I suggest that you put your phone and computer in a drawer at the same time every evening so you can unplug from technology well before bedtime. Experts in human behavior have found that being successful at making healthy lifestyle choices is less about motivation or willpower and more about setting up your life in a way that makes these decisions easier, so using these tools can make it easier to find more hours to sleep.

2. Create an optimal sleep environment.

Your bedroom should be your sleep sanctuary, and as long as you don't live in a studio apartment it should not double as your office, kitchen, or living room. You don't need expensive linens, a weighted blanket, or a cooling pad (although these are all nice); a comfortable mattress, a high-quality pillow, and soft bedding will do just fine. If you have indicator lights on electronics in your bedroom, cover them with black electrical tape. If you have bright streetlights outside your window, use blackout curtains. If you can hear traffic noise, use a white noise machine to drown it out. Finally, make sure your bedroom is nice and cool (the optimal temperature for sleeping is around sixty-five degrees).

You don't need an elaborate nighttime routine to improve your sleep, and most of us don't have the time for that anyway. Instead, focus on a "one-hour power-down." One hour before bed, shut down all electronics, including computers, tablets, and iPads. Put your phone in airplane mode except for emergency calls and use this time to get ready for sleep.

3. Calm your mind before bed.

Most insomnia is caused by ruminating about things that haven't happened and may never happen. The good news is that there are many ways to calm your mind and body for sleep. Experiment with the suggestions below and stick with what works for you.

- Journal before bed. Processing your worries by writing them down has been found to help clear the mind of stressful thoughts so they won't keep you up at night. Gratitude journaling is another way to send yourself to bed in a positive mind-set. Just setting aside a few minutes to write down three things that you are grateful for every evening is an easy and effective way to do this.
- Do some breathing exercises. If you're in an anxious or worried state, or just a little amped up, you can engage your calming parasympathetic nervous system by doing a few minutes of breathwork. I use the four-seven-eight breath technique I learned from Dr. Andrew Weil. Here's how to do it: Sitting calmly, place the tip of your tongue on the roof of your mouth near the back of your upper front teeth and breathe out with a *whoosh* sound. Then inhale through your nose to a silent count of four seconds, hold your breath for a count of seven, and breathe out through your mouth for a count of eight. Repeat this cycle three more times, for a total of four rounds. This technique has been clinically proven to help you relax your body and mind, and it takes just a few minutes!

The three tips above are necessary if you want to have a healthy sleep life. If you've already ticked those three off the list, you can turn to the following tips and tricks from your new Sleep Toolkit as well.

4. Experiment with magnesium.

Magnesium is often referred to as the "relaxation" mineral, thanks to its ability to combat stress, insomnia, anxiety, and muscle pain and tension. You can always take a magnesium supplement, but one of my favorite ways to use magnesium for sleep is by taking a warm bath with Epsom salts. Magnesium sulfate is the main component of Epsom salts, and by penetrating your skin and muscles it can have a relaxing effect. Even just soaking in a warm bath helps you fall asleep faster.[26] It's also difficult to text or watch TV from the bath, so it kills two birds with one stone.

5. Use aromatherapy.

Several studies have shown that essential oils can improve sleep quality and decrease anxiety.[27] [28] I love using an essential oil diffuser with a mix of lavender and other relaxing essential oils such as bergamot and ylang-ylang. These are inexpensive and really make your room smell amazing. You can also use an essential oil spray on your pillow if a diffuser feels like too much of a production.

6. Do some easy stretching.

Doing some stretching or restorative yoga before bed can help with pain, elevated blood pressure, restless leg syndrome, and anxiety. Even a few poses right before bed can engage your parasympathetic nervous system and help you sleep better.[29] I love doing legs-up-the-wall pose, child's pose, or even just savasana.

The best part is that you only need five or so minutes to make a big difference.

7. Try a cup of herbal tea.

One of my favorite ways to promote healthy sleep is by drinking an herbal tea with relaxing or sleep-inducing properties. This is best done a couple of hours before bed, so that you don't wake up to urinate in the middle of the night. Pick herbal teas with valerian root, chamomile, lemon balm, hops, or passionflower.[30] [31] Some of my favorites are Nighty Night Tea by Traditional Medicinals and Bedtime Tea by Yogi.

8. Wear blue-light-blocking glasses.

Wearing blue-light-blocking glasses is another supersimple way to revamp your sleep. And given the excessive amounts of melatonin-suppressing blue light in our homes, these are an essential in my house. Nighttime lenses are usually amber or orange and block out more than 90 percent of blue-spectrum light. Wearing blue-light-blocking glasses has been shown to significantly improve sleep quality and decrease insomnia.[32] My favorites are Swanwick glasses, but there are several good manufacturers, and prescription options as well. You can also change your CFL or incandescent lightbulbs to low-blue-light bulbs. There are several on the market—in fact, one of my patients invented a lightbulb called the Bedtime Bulb, which blocks out almost all blue- and green-spectrum light and lasts for several years.

We've learned in this chapter just how big a role sleep plays in our overall immune health. In fact, I've had dozens of patients who have been able to make measurable improvements in their autoimmune condition, allergies, chronic inflammation, or weakened immune system simply by moving sleep up on their priority list. I purposefully put the sleep chapter first in the Immune Restoration Plan because honestly, I think it's the most important! You can exercise and eat well and control stress, but if you're not sleeping, your immune system won't be as healthy as it would be if you were getting your recommended eight hours.

I know that improving sleep is easier said than done. But here's the good news: The tips in the next few chapters will also improve your sleep. Sleep is often the first thing to get disrupted when our lifestyle is out of balance, because it's affected not just by our sleep habits but also by our exercise routine, our diet, and especially our stress levels—which brings us to our next chapter.

CHAPTER 6

Optimize Your Stress — the Good and the Bad

In the early 1990s, I graduated from college with a degree in biology. But like a typical postgrad, I wasn't at all clear on what I wanted to do with my life. I did know that I needed a job and time to figure out my future. I got a job as a lab technician at the prestigious Rockefeller University in New York City in the laboratory of Dr. Bruce McEwen. And while I didn't know it then, this experience would end up shaping my career for many years. Dr. McEwen was a giant in the field of neuroendocrinology, especially when it came to studying the effects of stress hormones on the brain. He even coined the term "allostatic load," something we know now as the wear and tear that stress takes on the body.[1]

I was assigned to an amazing team of scientists who concentrated on studying the effects of acute and chronic stress on the immune systems of rats. While I was naïvely pipetting away, running radioimmunoassays and trying not to break the high-speed ultracentrifuge, the emerging field of psychoneuroimmunology was gaining traction in the scientific world. What is psychoneuroimmunology, exactly? It's basically the study of how our psychological state changes our biochemistry, therefore molding our immune system and health outcomes. This concept was relatively novel at the time, but over the past thirty years, research on how chronic stress shapes our immune system and hence human disease has exploded. In fact, this truth permeates how we think about immunity entirely. I left the lab after three years and found my way down to medical school in New Orleans, but my time at Rockefeller University influenced my path as a physician, and, of course, it helps shape this chapter, which is all about stress and the immune system.

THE MODERN "FIGHT-OR-FLIGHT" RESPONSE PROBLEM

Almost everyone I talk to has heard about the fight-or-flight response, and certainly all of us have felt it in our bodies at some point. It's that surge of adrenaline that causes your heart to race and triggers that nervous butterfly feeling in your stomach. Sometimes it's for a good reason—say, you're about to get married or accept an award in front of a crowd—but other times it's for not-so-great reasons, like receiving devastating news or realizing that someone is following you down a dark street at night. Either way, this stress response has been evolutionarily crucial to our survival as creatures on the planet. Like it or not, our stress response keeps us alive, protecting us from danger and giving us an instant hit of quick energy to fend off and/or run away from danger.

Let's just say, for example, that you step off a curb and narrowly miss being hit by a speeding bus. Instantly, the amygdala in your brain senses a threat to your safety, and within milliseconds your sympathetic nervous system is activated and two hormones—norepinephrine and epinephrine—pour into your circulation from nerve endings and your adrenal glands. These hormones increase your heart rate, dilate your pupils, shunt blood to your large muscles, and stimulate the release of glucose into the bloodstream so you can fight or flee. Shortly after this initial system is engaged, a second system, the hypothalamic-pituitary-adrenal (HPA) axis, is activated. This starts with a hormonal signal from the hypothalamus called corticotropin-releasing hormone (CRH), which travels to the pituitary gland nestled at the base of the brain. The pituitary gland then sends another hormonal signal, called adrenocorticotropic hormone (ACTH), which tells the adrenal glands sitting on top of the kidneys to pump out cortisol. This all takes just a few minutes, and if the stressor goes away, the parasympathetic nervous system activates a "relaxation response" that brings you back into balance. This is often called the "rest and digest" phase, because when you're having a stress response and cortisol surge, your ability to digest and sleep goes right out the window.

So what's the issue with stress, then? If our stress response is a beneficial evolutionary adaptation, why do we hear experts warn us about the "dangers of stress" all the time? Well, what experts are warning us about is not a short-term acute fight-or-flight response that quickly resolves like the bus example I just gave; they're warning us about the dangers of chronic, sustained stress, which has known negative effects on our health, including increasing the incidence of or worsening diseases like cancer,[2] heart disease,[3] depression,[4] and autoimmune disease.[5] Thousands of years ago, we had to deal with a ton of short-term stressors, like hunting for food, finding shelter, tribal warfare, and attacks by wild animals. (Makes our twenty-first-century life sound quite peachy,

doesn't it?) These days, stress comes in many sizes, shapes, and flavors, and unlike the bus incident, most of them—like arguments
with your spouse, work stress, getting stuck in traffic, and financial issues—are not immediately life-threatening. But here's the
tricky part: Our body registers these stressors in the same way as a
tiger approaching us in the jungle or a bus almost mowing us
down. And when you add up all these small stressors that are constantly triggering our fight-or-flight response, it leads to changes
in our immune system and disease state over time.

The reality is that the way stress affects our body comes down
to how we perceive the stress, how intense it is, and how long
we've been dealing with it. Unfortunately, our modern lives are
the perfect recipe for constant activation of the stress response.
Think about it: Most of us would say we're "under a lot of stress,"
but if you think about it, it's probably not really the stressor itself
that's doing the damage to our body; it's our body's sustained
physical and hormonal reaction that causes changes to our immune
system. Whether we perceive or imagine stress (yes, I'm talking to
all you worrywarts out there!) or actually experience physical or
psychological stress, the same reaction occurs in the body. As we
learned earlier, part of this has to do with the release of norepinephrine, epinephrine, CRH, and ACTH, but it also has to do
with cortisol, a hormone you've probably heard about once or
twice.

Cortisol often gets a bad rap in the wellness world, mostly
because people only talk about its negative effects. But the truth is
that just like the fight-or-flight response itself, we can't survive
without it! In fact, we secrete it all day long in a nice circadian
pattern, which is regulated by the "master clock" we learned
about in Chapter 5. When you look at the daily release of cortisol,
it's almost exactly opposite to that of melatonin. It goes like this:
Cortisol peaks around 7 a.m., helping us get ready to take on the

challenges of the day. Then it declines until it reaches its nadir around midnight. (That is, unless you're watching the eleven o'clock news in your bedroom or having a stressful late-night argument.) It then starts to slowly rise again until we open our eyes. Since cortisol rises and falls in this predictable pattern throughout the day, to get an accurate measurement of it, you have to test it at different times. In my practice I use home cortisol urine testing that can capture levels four or more times during the day and evening. This is crucial because even though your cortisol may be normal at one point during the day, it may be really low or high at other times and you wouldn't know it.

Cortisol Testing Options

Cortisol testing is very important in my medical assessments of patients. Many people come in with weight gain, immune issues, and fatigue, and I want to see whether their cortisol production is too low or too high due to chronic stress and dysfunction of their HPA axis. To do this I need to know what their levels are before they go to sleep and when they first roll out of bed. Testing is available to most people through standard laboratories, but it's impossible to accurately capture the ups and downs of cortisol throughout the day unless you decide to camp out at the lab and get multiple blood draws. Another way to measure cortisol is through home saliva or urine tests. These are both good choices, but urine testing has the advantage of looking at how you metabolize or break down cortisol, which can be helpful information. Most functional medicine practitioners can order and interpret these tests; however, they're generally not covered by insurance plans.

Cortisol wears many hats, ranging from helping regulate blood pressure, heart rate, and blood sugar to activating the immune system and the anti-inflammatory response. The fact that cortisol is anti-inflammatory may surprise you, but here's a connection that might help you make sense of it. Steroid drugs, such as prednisone, are akin to the medication form of cortisol and are used to decrease inflammation and cause immune suppression. Think about it: People get steroids injected into their knees for arthritis, spray steroids up their nose for allergies, take steroid pills for asthma flares, and rub cortisone cream on their skin for poison ivy. These are all ways that corticosteroid hormones, which include cortisol, are used to dampen the immune system response. What makes our cortisol response so complex is that depending on the timing, the frequency, and the amount of cortisol, the effects on our immune system are totally different. This is important because cortisol is a major contributing factor to the four Immunotypes.

STRESS: THE ACUTE AND THE CHRONIC

As we've seen a few times in this book already, oversimplifying the role of cortisol and flatly labeling it "bad" or "good" is not really accurate. Well, the same is true for stress as a whole. Dr. Firdaus Dhabhar, my former colleague and a renowned researcher in the field of positive and negative stress, devised a stress spectrum delineating how certain types of stress can be beneficial to our immune health and overall wellness.[6] Surprising, right? It will be less shocking when you think about the fact that a short-term acute stressor—like the bus incident—is designed to help your body supercharge all of its protective mechanisms in an instant. Because of this, acute stress actually helps boost your immune system in the short term. On the other end of the spectrum, Dr. Dhabhar teaches us that chronic stress can be bad news, causing immune dysregulation and immune suppression, leading to increased infections and poor recovery from diseases. We also know that frequent episodes of stress seem to exacerbate autoimmune diseases like rheumatoid arthritis[7] and ulcerative colitis[8] and can cause flare-ups in allergic reactions like eczema[9] and asthma.[10]

Here's the good news: Knowing what makes stress good or bad allows you to take critical steps to change your response to stress and create behaviors that protect you. All you have to do is learn how to promote good stress and cut down on the bad kind. Going back to the concept of allostatic load, you want to keep a balance of good stress and bad stress, which, let's be honest, none of us can avoid entirely. If you don't keep this balance, your immune system can dip into the dangerous territory of immune suppression, autoimmune reactions, inflammation, and worsening allergies.

Let's start with the good stress! As we just learned, acute stress may be good for you. When your body initially goes into a fight-or-flight situation, it senses a possibility that you might get wounded. Because of this, your white blood cells, such as neutrophils, natural killer cells (NK cells), and macrophages, redistribute from your circulation and make their way to areas like your skin, lungs, and GI tract so that they can take on any attack from the outside. Dr. Dhabhar likened this to soldiers moving from their barracks to the front lines or to different "battle stations," such as lymph nodes, to get ready to fight. It's not just cortisol that causes this effect; the other stress hormones, epinephrine and norepinephrine, are crucial in activating this acute immune response too.[11] So what qualifies as "good stress"? Well, things like intermittent fasting, cold showers, and working to meet an important academic goal are all great examples. But the best kind of good stress is exercise.

Exercise is a perfect example of how positive acute stress can benefit the immune system. If you exercise moderately for thirty to sixty minutes, there will be significant increases in your body of circulating immunoglobulins, neutrophils, NK cells, cytotoxic T cells, and macrophages.[12] This level of exercise is key for honing our immune function for things like improved surveillance of cancer cells[13] and decreasing inflammation[14] over time, not to mention the cardiovascular, metabolic, and mood-enhancing effects that exercise has on our bodies. In women, better responses to the flu vaccine were seen in studies when they either cycled for forty-five minutes or completed a tough mental task before the injection.[15] Epidemiological evidence indicates[16] that regular exercise reduces the incidence of many chronic diseases in older age, including infectious diseases from viruses and bacteria; cancers of the breast, colon, and prostate;[17] and chronic inflammatory diseases like heart disease.[18] In other words, exercise and short-term stress decrease inflammation and boost overall health. Recent studies have even shown that exercise can help improve recovery from COVID-19 infection.[19]

Now, on to the bad. Bad stress is a completely different ball of wax, and even low-level daily unrelenting stress has deleterious effects.[20] That's a problem because many of us don't have a great work-life balance. Chronic stress is linked to higher likelihood of metabolic syndrome, characterized by obesity, high blood pressure, insulin resistance, and high triglycerides. As we know, all of this ups your risk for heart attacks, diabetes, and strokes. In fact, people with chronic work stress were twice as likely to have metabolic syndrome as those without work stress.[21] A study of more than 600,000 men and women in Europe, the US, and Japan suggests that people with significant job stress and long work hours have a 10 to 40 percent greater risk of coronary heart disease than those without high stress![22] Yes, you can partially blame your job for your health issues. Chronic stress also messes with our cell-mediated immunity, which has a huge impact on surveillance and destruction of cancer cells. Chronic stress has been shown to increase the incidence of cancer, such as squamous cell skin cancer,[23] and may factor into increased spread of the disease.[24] Chronic stress can also increase the risk of autoimmune disease in those predisposed. In one study of 120,572 active military personnel with diagnosed post-traumatic stress disorder (PTSD), there was a 52 percent risk of developing autoimmune disease over five years.[25] Pretty astounding, isn't it?

Even stress early in life, both psychological and physical, can leave an imprint on our immune system. Adverse childhood events (ACEs) impact health later in life by changing how our immune system responds to stress in adulthood. This is a hot area of research, and one study revealed that in adult men and women with autoimmune disease, the incidence of at least one ACE was 64 percent, and the more traumatic childhood stress they reported, the higher the hospitalization rate for their disease.[26] It's clear that stress and the effects of cortisol and other stress hormones on our immune system are not so cut-and-dried. We can't say stress is all "bad," because in certain situations it's adaptive, necessary, and even positive. It all comes down to the chronicity, timing, and intensity of the stressor. And the way our brain perceives stress can change our biologic response. Some of us are genetically wired to withstand and deal with stress better, but it's a skill that the rest of us can hone with practice.[27] How? By working to build *resilience,* which is really the ability to adapt well in the face of challenges, adversity, trauma, and tragedy.

Stanford psychologist Kelly McGonigal writes in her book *The Upside of Stress* that people who see stress as a challenge and just part of life fare better healthwise than those who fear and avoid stress. Better resilience is attainable for all of us, and there are many ways to build resilience as well as manage your body's reactions to stressful events. The habits and lifestyle practices featured in the Toolkit below, if incorporated over time, will strengthen your resilience muscle. In addition, a myriad of natural substances that I will review can soften the blow stress strikes on your brain and subsequently your immune system. So while none of us can avoid all forms of negative stress, we have a lot more control over them than you've been led to believe!

YOUR STRESS TOOLKIT

Many of the recommendations below will substantially improve your stress response and make you more resilient in the face of daily stressors. However, improving your stress response requires daily attention, and for many of us who have created deep grooves in the pathway toward a fight-or-flight reaction, this may take time and practice. Prioritizing sleep still remains my number one tip for a better immune system, but practicing stress management is a close second. The good news is that better sleep will result in lower stress, and lower stress will help you sleep better. This is what I like to call a positive snowball effect—where improving one aspect of your health automatically jump-starts other aspects of healing.

So, without further ado, here are just some of the interventions to help you tackle stress head-on, feel calmer and more resilient, and lower your risk of stress-related diseases.

1. Create a daily mindfulness practice.

I know, I know. You've heard this before! I'd bet my life savings that the majority of you have tried (and failed) to establish a regular meditation practice. As a doctor who frequently recommends meditation to my patients, I hear "I don't have time!" "I can't sit still!" and "My mind just starts racing when I try!" over and over again. If you've thought of a million reasons why you can't meditate, let me say this: You will not become a meditation master or Buddhist monk overnight—or realistically, ever. And here's the thing—that's totally fine! Mindfulness is way more than meditation; in fact, you don't even have to sit still or clear your mind to reap the benefits. There are many ways to be mindful, and the data showing how beneficial they are to our health and immune system is mind-blowing. In fact, regular mindfulness meditation lowers inflammation markers like IL-6, NF-κB, and CRP while strengthening our cell-mediated immunity.[28]

I always recommend starting with something as simple as a body scan, where you progressively relax each part of your body while lying on the floor or your bed. If that's too hard, you can just listen to guided meditation and follow the instructions. If sitting still is too hard, you can do a walking meditation, which is popular in several forms of Buddhism. You just focus deliberately on the movements with each step and on your breathing while you walk. It's the most relaxing walk you've ever done! I recommend aiming for at least ten minutes a day. There are numerous apps, too, many of them free, that provide thousands of options. My favorite apps are Calm, InsightTimer, Headspace, and Breethe. The key is to start where you are and "practice" daily. You may never get to a place where meditation feels seamless and easy— and that's okay! You'll get the benefits just the same.

2. Take a digital detox once a month.

This is one of my favorite ways to decrease stress. All you have to do is take one day a month and turn off all access to social media, news, email, and TV. Use this time to get outside, read a book (a printed one), cook, exercise, play with your pets and enjoy face-to-face interactions with your friends and family. I promise you, you'll feel calmer and less stressed, and even though it's just one day a month, you'll reap the benefits for weeks. In fact, you may love the feeling so much that you decide to do it more frequently!

3. Monitor your thoughts.

Cognitive behavioral therapy (CBT) is a method used by psychologists and mental health professionals to help with anxiety, depression, addiction, and many other mental health and even physical health issues. And here's a secret: You don't need to see a therapist to take advantage of CBT. In fact, you can use it on yourself to help manage your responses to stressful events. We tend to be wired to have a knee-jerk reaction to stressors; this response can be so automatic that our rational brain doesn't have a chance to actually process what's going on. For example: Do you always honk your horn and curse when someone cuts you off on the road? Does your mind always go to the worst-case scenario when your phone rings? Do you assume someone is mad at you if they don't smile or say hello? If you answered yes to any or all of these questions, you're not alone.

There's a useful CBT exercise called the Think-Feel-Act Cycle that can halt these knee-jerk reactions and allow us to think about our emotions and feelings before acting. Here's how to try it out: The next time you feel an emotion in your body such as fear, worry, or anger, trace it back to the original thought you had in your brain. Maybe it's "I gave a bad presentation and I'm going to be fired" or "People will always let you down." Then, really think about where that thought came from, and more important, *ask yourself if it's really true.* Oftentimes, you find that it's not true at all. This may seem like a small change, but this exercise can transform your feelings about the situation and, therefore, your reaction to it as well. Over time, you'll feel more in control, more positive, happier, and less at the mercy of the stressful events around you.

4. Get outside.

Imagine if you went to your doctor and instead of prescribing a drug for what ails you, the doctor gave you a prescription for "nature." Well, studies have shown that being outside in nature can dial down your stress and calm your stress response in a major way.[29] In fact, being out in nature can lower your cortisol and lessen perceived feelings of worry while increasing joy. Immersing yourself in nature has also been found to improve immune function. There are many ways to do this. You can take a walk in your local park, go to the beach, meander through a garden, or hike in a state park—focus on going anywhere you can escape from technology, traffic, and noise for a while and see something green!

5. Move your body daily.

As I've mentioned, exercise is the ultimate form of positive stress. And ironically, it's also one of the best ways to increase resilience and decrease negative stress! Studies show that regular light and moderate aerobic exercise can decrease cortisol and adrenaline levels over time while increasing the release of pleasurable endorphins in the brain. In addition, exercise can help alleviate depression and anxiety.[30] This is especially true when it comes to restorative movement like tai chi, yoga, stretching, and walking, which lower stress hormones while also subjectively improving mood.

Endurance exercise and high-intensity interval training (HIIT) will increase cortisol temporarily, and they're fantastic for your metabolism, mood, and cardiovascular health. Just make sure you have enough recovery time or restorative workouts between sessions.[31] Cortisol is a catabolic hormone—that is, it breaks down muscle and fat—and if it floods your body without time to recover, you may be setting yourself up for injury.[32] Studies have shown that the cortisol elevations that occur with long, intense runs can take up to forty-eight hours to return to a normal baseline.[33] Marathon participants who pound the pavement for 26.2 miles have high markers of oxidative stress and higher levels of inflammation. Overtraining syndrome, which is characterized by lowered immunity, fatigue, and mood changes, is thought to be caused partially by the disruption of a normal cortisol feedback response, as well as the tanking of other hormones, like testosterone.[34] Well-known American marathoner Ryan Hall retired from competitive running at the young age of thirty-three, citing debilitating fatigue and depression caused by overtraining. Don't get me wrong, I am a huge fan of endurance exercise and intense workouts, having completed a few marathons and triathlons myself. But I've also been on the receiving end of some pretty awful fatigue and adrenal imbalance when I didn't complement these activities with proper sleep and stress management. Depending on your Immunotype and your current health, there may be times when intense exercise is not the best option for you.

6. Try adaptogens.

Although I've covered the most important things you can do to manage stress and balance the effects of cortisol on the immune system, there are natural substances called adaptogens that through their effects on the neurohormonal systems of the body, can counteract the destructive effects of chronic stress, increase energy and cardiovascular endurance, and decrease anxiety.[35] These plant pharmaceuticals were first used by Russian soldiers in World War II to increase stamina and endurance, but were also tested out by explorers of the Arctic, astronauts heading off into space, and others in situations that create intense mental and physical stress. Although each adaptogen works slightly differently, their goal in the body is to provide energy and resilience, protect the brain and nervous system, or calm and reduce the effects of excess stress. Some adaptogens are balancing and some are energizing, so depending on the way your cortisol levels and stress response are acting, you may need a specific type of adaptogen. Some of the most studied and effective adaptogens are:

- **Rhodiola rosea**—Rhodiola is a root that grows naturally in Europe, Asia, and North America; it has been studied extensively for stress management.[36]
- **Eleuthero (Siberian ginseng)**—Ginseng is a small, woody shrub native to northeastern Asia that has been studied for a variety of health benefits.[37]
- **Schisandra**—Schisandra is a berry that grows in northern China and Korea and has well-known anti-stress effects.[38]
- **Ashwagandha**—Ashwagandha is an herb that has been used for centuries in traditional Indian medicine to reduce stress and enhance well-being.[39]

- **Panax ginseng**—This energizing herb has been used in traditional Chinese and Korean medicine to help with a wide range of health issues.[40]

- **Lemon balm**—This fresh, fragrant herb is in the same family as mint and has historically been used for culinary and medicinal purposes. It has also been used for anxiety and to improve cognition.[41]

- **Magnolia bark**—Magnolia bark is just what the name suggests, a medicinal preparation made from the bark, leaves, and flowers of the magnolia tree. It has been shown to help induce relaxation and lower perceived stress.[42]

I'll be talking more about adaptogens and other natural substances that are useful in regulating our stress when we get into each Immunotype, and you'll see how these magical substances can create a more balanced immune profile.

Getting a handle on stress and getting great sleep are the foundations of a healthy immune system. Without sleep and stress management, the rest of the advice in this book will only be marginally helpful. Even adopting just one of these lifestyle changes will go a long way toward helping to reverse autoimmune disease, strengthening a weak immune system, decreasing chronic inflammation that's been festering for years, and restoring balance to an out-of-whack immune response.

CHAPTER 7

Tend to Your GALT—the Home of Your Immune System

For ten years I worked as an allergist in private practice, and 100 percent of my patients came in with some sort of allergic or immune problem. Looking back, I see that I never once inquired or even thought about their gut health. Now it's one of the first things I evaluate. It's taken a few centuries of research and discovery for us to understand the importance of this gut-immune relationship, but if there's one thing that becomes clearer to me every single day, it's that your gut is the epicenter of your immune system. This might seem strange to you. Why would your immune cells hang out there? Aren't they supposed to be circulating through the bloodstream and lymphatic pathways scanning for danger, or hanging out in peripheral lymph nodes of your body waiting to be called to duty? The reality is that most of these cells can be found at your immune system's central intelligence center—also referred to as the gut-associated lymphoid tissue, or GALT.[1] This is something we've known intuitively for hundreds of years—Hippocrates, the father of modern medicine, is well known for saying "All disease begins in the gut." But we lacked the advanced technology to really understand it. These days, however, we know that GALT is a cluster of lymph tissue that contains the highest concentration of immune cells in the entire body. Lining the small and large intestine, this tissue contains huge collections of B cells, T cells, macrophages, and dendritic cells. Scientific papers cite that approximately 70 percent of our total immune cells reside in the GALT,[2] about one cell layer away from the inside of our intestinal tract.

When you think about it, it makes a lot of sense that the gut would be the center of our immune system. Why? Because the gut is where we interact with most foreign substances—both friendly and dangerous. The gut is where we sample the world— all the substances we eat, drink, swallow, and to a certain extent even breathe will find their way down through our esophagus, through our stomach, and eventually into our vast intestinal tract, where our immune cells have to make decisions on what to do with everything. In a manner of speaking, the insides of our intestines are outside our body—that is, the cells that make up the barrier wall of our intestines (along with the thick mucous layer) are what separates the "outside world" from our bloodstream and the internal world of our body. This means that the microbes, food, toxins, and everything else that ends up in the intestinal tube pass right by ground zero of the immune system. Our intestinal cells create tight junctions with each other to prevent pathogens, food particles, and other substances from crossing this barrier willy-nilly; our dendritic cells can also extend their starfish-like arms across this barrier to sample the substances passing by. They're performing their job of immune surveillance and reconnaissance to decide what is friend or foe.

I mentioned that dendritic cells are part of our innate immune response, but they are also the couriers that take pieces of antigens back to T cells so they can decide what to do with that information—for instance, whether they need to send out cytokines, tell B cells to make antibodies, or do nothing. Dendritic cells are constantly dipping their fingers into the gut to figure out what's going on. Other specialized macrophages called M cells can engulf bacteria in the intestines and take them back to the lymph nodes for inspection too. Plasma cells can also pump IgA into the intestines, where it can glom onto dangerous bacteria and viruses that make their way into the gut, thereby protecting us from invasion.

So much activity! Pretty amazing that all this is happening within this thin barrier inside the body, isn't it? You can think of this area like Customs and Border Protection—it's where the body tries to prevent anything dangerous from slipping across its borders to wreak havoc on the inside. The other, even more important reason why our immune system is clustered so close to the gut is because it needs to be near our gut microbiota.

MEET YOUR MICROBIAL ALLIES

More commonly referred to as the gut microbiome, the gut microbiota is a collection of bacteria, fungi, archaea (an ancient single-celled microorganism), viruses, and parasites with an overall population of about 38 trillion organisms. Yes, that's a lot of microbes residing inside you! In fact, in a recent article in the journal *Nature,* it was determined that humans are about 50 percent human cells and 50 percent microbial cells. It's mind-blowing.[3] We truly are interspecies organisms with a supercomplex ecosystem. And without this universe of microorganisms, the human race would be toast. The microbial inhabitants in our gut do so many essential tasks for us, from breaking down fiber and creating fuel, to feeding and repairing our cells, to synthesizing B vitamins and other nutrients, to helping protect and develop our immune system and shielding us from dangerous invaders.[4]

About 1,000 species of bacteria have already been identified as inhabitants of the human gut, but on average, most of us have about 160 different ones in our gut at any one time. Unfortunately, as we age, many of us lose beneficial diversity because of antibiotics, prescription drugs, and poor diets, leading to an imbalanced or "dysbiotic" microbiota.[5] This is not good news for us, considering the fact that most of our gut bacteria are beneficial and we've evolved alongside them for thousands of years. (In other words: We need them!) Some scientists have even called the microbiome collectively "a forgotten organ."[6] If you're reading this and thinking "But wait, I thought bacteria were dangerous! Isn't our immune system there to protect us from them?" you're not alone. In recent years, we've launched a full-blown attack on germs with antibacterial soaps, hand sanitizers, and the overuse of antibiotics and antimicrobial medications. And while there are some not-so-friendly bugs in the community—like parasites, certain viruses, and problematic bacteria like *Clostridium difficile*—most of the bacteria are helpful, and the diversity of good bacteria in the gut is one of the major things that keep the bad guys in check. Therefore, when we disrupt our microbiome balance, we put ourselves at risk for opportunistic bugs to come in and wreck the place.

BACTERIA AS OUR TEACHERS

Two-year-old toddlers spend their days learning basic commands, simple words, and how to get from crawling to walking. However, they're also curating their microbiome. The first thousand days of human life are the most crucial when it comes to establishing a healthy microbiome.[7] We pick up vaginal and skin flora at birth, and these bacteria become the first inhabitants of our GI tract. Along the way, we also take in microbes from food, antibodies from breast milk if we're lucky enough to be breastfed, and organisms when we play in the dirt, with pets and our playmates. That's why the use of broad-spectrum antibiotics and the overuse of antimicrobial soap early in life can be disruptive and can increase the risk for immune issues like allergies and autoimmune disease later on in life. When we're babies, our immune system tolerates all these new beneficial bacteria, allowing them to seed our gut instead of creating an inflammatory reaction to them.[8] This is partly how we establish immune tolerance to normal everyday things like pollen and peanuts. In fact, in the absence of these bacteria, we cannot create a robust immune system. This was seen most clearly in experiments done in germ-free mice. These mice, which were bred without any intestinal bacteria, were found to have small, underdeveloped lymph nodes and reduced numbers of helper T cells, as well as fewer IgA-producing plasma cells. Basically, without friendly bacteria, the mice's immune systems were visibly abnormal.

Other studies have shown that a certain bacterium in our gut called *Bacteroides fragilis* changes how our immune system develops. It goes like this: Let's say a dendritic cell picks up and delivers this friendly bacterium back to the lymph nodes, where it gets presented to a helper T cell.[9] Instead of an inflammatory response, this causes both a shift in cytokines and a change in the type of helper T cells produced, resulting in an increase of regulatory T cells, which balance and calm the immune system, and a decrease in Th2 cells, which are responsible for allergies, asthma, and eczema. This may be one of the reasons why children who grow up on farms and in environments where they have a wider exposure to different bacterial and fungal organisms have been found to have lower incidence of asthma later on in life.[10]

The bacteria living in the gut are also crucial in creating tolerance to our own tissues. Remember, our immune system has to be able to tell the good guys from the bad guys, food from toxin, and damaged cells from healthy ones. That way, we can digest and absorb nutrients without launching an inflammatory response against them, but still maintain our ability to keep out the harmful stuff. How do these friendly bacteria do this? All bacteria can communicate with one another through "quorum sensing," which allows them to transmit messages about their immediate environment and then change their gene expression in response to what they sense.[11] Bacteria in the gut have turf wars with dangerous pathogens, competing with them for space, food, and oxygen and even changing the pH levels in your gut, as if they're forcing them out by sucking all the air out of the room.[12] This amazing ability of our commensal—or friendly, native bacteria—to manipulate the environment of the microbiome to fight infections is one of the reasons why fermented foods are so good for gut health. For example, *Lactobacillus* species, which are key beneficial bacteria found in humans, are also found naturally in yogurt and sauerkraut, as well as in commercial probiotics.

As you can see, a healthy and diverse gut microbiome is essential for excellent long-term health; unfortunately, a weakened microbiome—something that has become more and more widespread—does just the opposite.

WHAT YOUR GUT IS TELLING YOU

Unfortunately, we don't always get a telegram from our gut bacteria telling us that something is off. We expect at least some

rumbling, diarrhea, gas, or bloat to give us the heads-up. Sometimes that is the case, but more often than not a breakdown in the
gut microbiome doesn't show up this way. Instead we get food
allergies, asthma, autoimmune issues, or brain diseases like Parkinson's or Alzheimer's.[13] [14] All four Immunotype imbalances can
be triggered by dysfunction in the gut. For example, toxins that
we ingest can elicit an inflammatory response, leading to a Smoldering Immunotype; overgrowth of pathogenic bacteria can trigger autoimmune reactions and a Misguided Immunotype; chronic
stress can create a leaky gut-immune barrier and a Hyperactive
Immunotype; and a deficit of healthy microbes can lead to a Weak
Immunotype. So it's paramount to restore a healthy and robust
microbiome and efficient GALT.

That said, sometimes we do get gut symptoms that alert us
that something is going on. This is clearly the case in inflammatory bowel disease (IBD), which is an umbrella term used for a
group of autoimmune digestive diseases that includes Crohn's disease and ulcerative colitis. IBS affects more than 6.8 million people the world over, with higher rates in the US and Northern
Europe. And although genetic susceptibilities exist, diet and environmental factors that change the microbiome and impair immune
system functioning are key triggers.[15] For example, Western diets
high in animal and trans fats can increase inflammation by pro-
moting harmful bacterial endotoxins and dysbiosis in the gut.[16] A
particularly nasty *E. coli* strain—adherent-invasive *E. coli* (AIEC)—
found in Crohn's disease patients is thought to possibly provoke
the disease.[17] Pathogens like this and others can trigger the presence of Th17 cells, which increase intestinal inflammation and
play a role in many autoimmune diseases. (In IBD patients, it's
common to find a lot of Th17 cells in ulcerated areas.)[18]

Now that you know this, it won't come as a big shock to learn
that gut bacterial imbalance instigates other autoimmune diseases.

Rheumatoid arthritis is associated with elevations in the bacterial genus *Prevotella*,[19] as well as a higher incidence of infection with the Epstein–Barr virus. However, it's not just the bad bugs that might trigger autoimmune disease; it's also the loss of healthy flora that act as "gut guardians." Low counts of a protective bacterium called *Faecalibacterium prausnitzii* are found in Crohn's disease and ankylosing spondylitis,[20] an arthritis that primarily affects younger men. In patients with psoriasis, decreased diversity and low levels of *Akkermansia* and *Ruminococcus* bacteria have been seen.[21] Overall, it's clear that a messed-up gut microbiome drives autoimmune disease, by way of an increase in pathogens stimulating inflammation, but also because of a dearth of protective species.

Gut microbes are also superinfluencers when it comes to major diseases like cardiovascular disease[22] and diabetes.[23] We've learned in recent years that a chemical called trimethylamine N-oxide (TMAO) slows down the removal of cholesterol from the body and increases the amount of atherosclerotic plaque in vessels, leading to many of these diseases. In fact, a high level of TMAO has been shown to be an independent predictor of both short-term and long-term major adverse cardiac events.[24] Turns out that meat-eaters produce more TMAO in their bodies, as their microbes break down a substance called choline found in meat and eggs, which then converts to TMAO in the liver. You've probably heard quite a few times that diets high in animal products can contribute to heart disease; well, this research suggests that the protein in animal products causing shifts in the microbiome and excess TMAO may explain this link. In fact, if you look at the microbiome makeup of vegans, vegetarians, and carnivores, the microbial fingerprint in the gut looks totally different. Yes, TMAO is bad, but that doesn't mean you have to eschew meat completely. And eating a 100-percent-plant-based diet doesn't guarantee that you'll have a happy gut, either. Read on.

LEAKY GUT AND YOUR IMMUNE SYSTEM

"Leaky gut" is a term that has been thrown around a lot in the past decade or so. In fact, a Google search of these two words yields 8,120,000 hits. Surprisingly, a lot of conventional doctors pooh-pooh this concept, despite mounting evidence that it's a real problem at the heart of many diseases. "Leaky gut" isn't a true medical term, but it basically means that you have increased intestinal permeability (and that is a mouthful). So what is leaky gut and how does it come about?

Many things can contribute to intestinal permeability, such as alcohol, toxins, medications, stress, intestinal infections, radiation, microbiome imbalances, and even some foods — really anything that can disrupt the protective microbiome, cause inflammation, and damage the delicate mucosal barrier between our gut and our bloodstream, which as we learned earlier is controlled by "tight junctions." When tight junctions become more permeable, they allow partially digested food particles, microbes, and chemicals to slip through to the GALT and the bloodstream. When this happens, your immune system has to deal with all these foreign substances that have "leaked" through, and the closely controlled system goes haywire, triggering cytokine activation and immune responses against foods and even "self-proteins," which can begin the cycle of autoimmune disease.

Dr. Alessio Fasano, a famed researcher in celiac disease and an expert on the gut barrier, explains that when there is disruption to the tight junctions, a substance called zonulin is involved.[25] Zonulin is secreted by the intestinal cells in response to bacteria like salmonella, but also in response to gluten, the protein found in wheat. You can think of zonulin as a doorman of sorts to the tight junctions in your GI tract, opening and closing the junctions as needed. When zonulin is high, the tight junctions stay open, leading to higher intestinal permeability.[26] Elevations in zonulin are characteristic of celiac disease but can also be seen in patients who have nonceliac gluten sensitivity.[27] When you have a leaky gut, it sets off a massive cycle of immune activation to all the substances slipping through the gut barrier. This causes major inflammation and can contribute to a long list of diseases. In fact, an elevation in zonulin—and hence leaky gut—is linked to diseases such as type 1 diabetes, multiple sclerosis, and asthma. Leaky gut is what connects gut microbial imbalance and disease, so if you want to reverse this cycle, you need to focus on eliminating the causes of gut microbial imbalances and reverse and heal your leaky gut.

Should You Get Your Microbiome Tested?

Although there are many direct-to-consumer tests that look into your microbiome and promise to tell you if there's an issue with your gut health, they vary in accuracy. It's best to work with a trained functional medicine practitioner who has experience deciphering these tests and helping people heal their gut. However, if you are interested in collecting your poop at home (yes, this is unfortunately part of the process!) and are curious about what you might find, there are several companies to choose from, such as Viome, BIOHM, and Thryve. Just be forewarned that these tests have their limitations and you'll often be urged to buy targeted supplements and probiotics with your report.

THE TOP GUT HEALTH SABOTEURS

When I broach the subject of gut health with my patients, it's not uncommon for them to respond by saying something along the lines of "But I came in for immune issues! My digestion is fine." But remember: You may have a gut problem even if you don't have classic GI problems like stomachaches, diarrhea, or bloating. In fact, symptoms like rashes, arthritis, depression, and brain fog can be a sign that you're dealing with a gut imbalance. People are often amazed at the dysfunction we find when we look a little closer at gut health. To find out how much your gut may be contributing to your immune system imbalance, ask yourself if any of the following apply to you:

- **Frequent or chronic use of antibiotics.** Even if you haven't taken antibiotics in years, oftentimes we forget about the chronic ear infections we had as a child, the antibiotics we took for acne as a teenager, or all the urinary tract infections and cases of sinusitis, bronchitis, or strep throat we've had throughout the years. Unfortunately, all antibiotic treatments lead to severely depleted good bacteria and allow for the overgrowth of unfriendly ones. In fact, *Clostridium difficile* infections, which kill thousands of people a year, are primarily caused by the use of broad-spectrum antibiotics, which make your gut vulnerable to this bacterium.[28] And here's the thing that will really get you: According to the CDC, at least 30 percent of these antibiotic prescriptions are completely unnecessary. (In my mind, that number is probably more like 50 or 60 percent!) The overprescription of antibiotics is a massive problem—and our guts and immune systems end up paying the price.

- **Traveler's diarrhea or food poisoning.** Anytime we get infected with a pathogenic bacterium, virus, or parasite, it causes not only inflammation but also imbalance in the gut. Bacterial infections like shigella, salmonella, and campylobacter (three very common gut infections acquired while traveling) can cause major issues with gut motility and sometimes months or years of chronic IBS symptoms. They are also autoimmune triggers.[29]

- **Chronic stress.** We talked in the previous chapter about the way cortisol can weaken the gut-immune barrier. Being lonely, depressed, or stressed affects your mucosal immunity directly by lowering the amount of IgA antibody your B cells make. Remember, IgA hangs out all along your gut lining as a first defense against invaders, so if you're constantly in a state of stress or feel overwhelmed, make sure you pay close attention to the advice in Chapter 6.

- **Lack of fiber.** Although many of us are obsessed with our fat-carb-protein ratios, an estimated 95 percent of us don't eat enough fiber![30] The consequences of this are severe, considering that high-fiber diets are associated with less obesity, less cancer, and less chronic disease. Fiber is important for our GALT because our friendly gut bugs thrive on fiber and resistant starches from plant foods.[31] You'll often hear fiber referred to as "prebiotics" because it essentially acts as food for the bacteria in our gut. Bacteria break down and ferment fiber to create an amazing substance called butyrate that's like rocket fuel for our cells, giving them energy and inducing autophagy (remember, we want more of that). Studies have shown that butyrate can help prevent colon cancer[32] and that it also lowers the pH level in the gut, making it less hospitable for certain bugs like pathogenic *E. coli.*

- **Glyphosate/genetically modified organism (GMO) foods.** Roundup is the most commonly used herbicide in the world and is used on genetically modified crops. The active ingredient glyphosate is known to disrupt the microbiome of lab animals, and one can only assume human microbiome species as well.[33] In 2015 the World Health Organization (WHO) also ruled that glyphosate was a carcinogen, so there's that, too.[34] The best way to avoid glyphosate is to avoid GMO foods as much as possible. Common glyphosate-contaminated foods include corn, oats, canola oil, soy, and potatoes.

Evaluating all of the above will give you an idea of what your risk factors might be for microbiome dysfunction and where you might land on the spectrum of gut health. Another factor I would keep in mind is your consumption of alcohol, which can injure the mucosal lining and muscle wall in the small intestine and allow toxins to pass more easily into the blood. Alcohol also kills bacteria, which is great in a hand sanitizer but not in your microbiome. Also take stock of how many times you pop NSAIDs like ibuprofen for pain. Despite being over-the-counter, these can cause damage and even ulceration of the GI tract if used too frequently.

YOUR GALT RESURRECTION TOOLKIT

The first thing I recommend to my patients who want to heal their gut is a thirty-day elimination diet that removes common gut irritants. This is truly the gold standard for diagnosing food sensitivities and intolerances, as standard food allergy testing will only reveal the foods to which you have an IgE or anaphylactic-type reaction. Many people have intolerances to foods they have difficulty digesting, such as lactose intolerance, or they may have sensitivities caused by having IgG antibodies against the foods themselves. This often shows up in milder symptoms that might be delayed for hours or even days, so it's extremely difficult to pinpoint which foods are the problematic ones. Although there are tests for diagnosing IgG-based food sensitivities, they vary in validity, are expensive, and are not covered by insurance. If you have the opportunity to do this kind of test with a health care provider trained in interpretation of the test's results, great, but first I recommend working with a nutritionist, registered dietitian, or integrative practitioner on an elimination diet.

If you're going it alone, I recommend removing what I see as the biggest sensitivities for most people—wheat, soy, dairy, eggs, and corn. I also have people remove any added sugars, caffeine, and alcohol for the first thirty days. Most people notice a huge difference in symptoms once they've eliminated these foods from their daily diet and are surprised that seemingly unrelated symptoms like skin rashes, joint aches, and headaches go away. Then you reintroduce each food one at a time, waiting at least forty-eight hours to ascertain whether any symptoms return. This is often when my patients notice trigger foods that may be giving them heartburn or GI distress; and it allows them to continue eating everything else so as not to eliminate foods unnecessarily. See Chapter 10 for more details on how to do an elimination diet.

In addition to an elimination diet, the following tips can help you heal from gut imbalances and leaky gut so that your microbiome starts working for you, not against you.

1. **Eat more plants:** We know that a diverse plant-based diet is the key to great gut health. And while that doesn't mean that you should never enjoy animal-based foods, your microbiome needs the fiber found in beans, whole

gluten-free grains, veggies, and fruit on a daily basis to be healthy. This will also increase the amount of gut-healing butyrate available in your colon. Aim for a minimum of 25 grams of fiber a day if you're a woman and 38 grams if you're a man. You can add extra fiber to salads and smoothies by including seeds and nuts, too.

2. **Incorporate fermented foods:** Fermentation has been used for eons as a way to preserve foods without refrigeration so that humans could eat fruits and vegetables all year long. Well, our ancestors were onto something, because fermentation of fruits and veggies, grains, and milks can also provide beneficial live probiotic organisms, like *Lactobacillus* and *Bifidobacterium,* that can help restore balance to the gut. Fermented foods are also easier to digest, may lower blood pressure, and contain beneficial antioxidants. Plenty of studies show that naturally occuring probiotics produce antimicrobial agents that suppress the growth of pathogenic organisms.[35] *Lactobacillus* can improve the integrity of the intestinal barrier, which helps in the immune tolerance needed for preventing autoimmune disease and allergies. But before you go stocking up on peach yogurt, know that many "probiotic" foods like conventional yogurt don't have any live cultures in them and instead are just filled with sugar. Instead, try fermented veggies like raw sauerkraut or spicy kimchi—even a tablespoon a day will help! The other benefit of eating fermented veggies is that your prebiotic fiber is already built in, so you get a two-for-one deal.

3. **Take a probiotic supplement:** If it's not realistic for you to eat fermented foods on a daily basis, probiotics are a great option, but they vary widely in quality. Always look for the Good Manufacturing Practice (GMP) and

U.S. Pharmacopeia (USP) stamp on the bottle, which guarantees that you're buying what the bottle claims. Probiotics should list all the species of bacteria and the numbers of each in colony-forming units (CFU) on the bottle, and unless otherwise noted, probiotics should always be refrigerated to guarantee viability. Most probiotic supplements will have multiple species of both *Bifidobacterium* and *Lactobacillus* bacteria, which are both native to the human microbiome. I recommend trying to get at least eight different species and a minimum of 30 billion CFU. Depending on your digestive needs, you may need a larger dose, but this is a good place to start. The higher the count and quality, the more expensive the probiotic, so you do get what you pay for.

I hope this chapter has convinced you of the fact that your gut microbiome is a critical part of your immune system. Unfortunately, our modern lifestyle puts our gut health to the test and often leaves us vulnerable to imbalances and leaky gut, which can set our immune system off in the wrong direction. The good news is that a few small changes in your life can make a big difference to your gut health.

CHAPTER 8

Toxins — The Ultimate Immune System Distracters

Your genes aren't your destiny, which is a good thing for some of us if maybe we weren't dealt the best hand. Of course, you inherit your DNA from your mom and dad, but how those genes play out over your lifetime has more to do with your environment. I've talked about our "environment" a few times already in this book. But what really defines our environments as humans? I'm not talking purely about the weather or the climate we live in. I'm talking about sleep, stress, the food we put into our body, and, most important, the substances that our bodies are exposed to every day. Think about it like this: Our genetics are the raw material of our body, and our environment is the sum total of everything that our body comes into contact with year after year, whether the quality of the air we breathe, the chemicals in the medications we take, the lotion we lather on our skin, or the water we drink.

So what does our environment have to do with our immune system? Well, we often make the mistake of thinking that the immune system is only for fighting infections when the truth is, it's also there to fend off foreign substances of all kinds—including toxins. "Toxins" is a word that's used all the time in the wellness world, so let me define it quickly before we discuss why they are so important to avoid. Some examples of toxins are:

- **Heavy metals,** like lead found in old paint or mercury found in some seafood.
- **Xenoestrogens,** which are chemicals found in certain products and foods that mimic estrogen.
- **Pesticides and herbicides,** which are used in nonorganic farming.
- **Plastics,** which contain chemicals like bisphenol A (BPA) that can leach out of the plastic and into the body.
- **Phthalates and parabens,** which are found in many cosmetics and personal care products.
- **Pharmaceutical drugs,** which contain foreign ingredients that can act as toxins that the body has to metabolize.
- **Fire-retardant chemicals,** which are found in mattresses, furniture, curtains, and some clothing.

Think about how often you use plastic, eat a nonorganic piece of food, use a lipstick or lotion, take a medication, drink tap water, or come in contact with any of the items on the list above—probably multiple times a day, right? Well, think about each tiny toxic exposure like a little fire that our immune system has to put out.

Knowing this, it's no surprise that toxins play a major role in creating our Immunotype. They can cause immune suppression and trigger autoimmune disease, allergies, and inflammation. This starts before birth and is a factor throughout our lives as our environments change for the better and for the worse. In fact, a well-known study done in 2004 found 287 chemicals in the umbilical cord blood of newborns! Of these chemicals, 180 were known carcinogens in humans or animals, 217 were neurotoxic, and 208 were known to cause birth defects.[1] So even before birth we're exposed to chemicals that our immune systems need to deal with.

As we go through our lives, this gets even worse. So many diseases we suffer from as adults have their roots in early life exposure to chemicals and toxins because they change our Immunotype from one that's balanced to one that is Smoldering, Misguided, Hyperactive, or Weak. This is partly because the immune system is still developing when we're infants, so it's particularly sensitive to chemicals.[2] However, even when we're adults, chemicals continue to have a major impact on our immune system health.

HOW CHEMICALS SABOTAGE OUR IMMUNE SYSTEM

The reality is that every day, we breathe in toxins, eat or drink them, or are exposed to them through our skin. That is literally life on planet Earth. How toxins affect our immune system on a cellular level is still a topic of active research, but already, study after study shows that:

- Toxins directly impair our immune cells, weakening our T cell response, macrophage activity, NK cell response, and antibody production.[3]
- Short-term exposure to cigarette smoke makes our macrophages less responsive to cytokines, essentially making them less effective.[4]
- Toxins cause problems by activating a receptor called AHR, which turns on genes that regulate enzymes in our liver detox pathways, causing liver damage, mutations to DNA, immune suppression, birth defects, and even tumors.[5]

- Phthalates, which are found in everything from shampoo, to soft, chewable baby toys, to PVC flooring, have been linked to wheezing and inflammatory health problems in children.[6]
- Hormone-disrupting chemicals that are sometimes referred to as "obesogens" promote the growth of fat cells, which contributes to metabolic syndrome.[7]
- Autoimmune diseases like rheumatoid arthritis and lupus have been linked to exposures to pesticides, mercury and lead, BPA, solvents, and certain medications.[8]
- Autoimmune diseases—such as primary biliary choloangitis (PBC), previously called primary biliary cirrhosis, and lupus—were found to be higher in women who used nail polish and hair dye.[9]

By now, hopefully, I've convinced you that toxins do play a significant role in all types of immune dysfunction, including the dysfunction seen in all four Immunotypes, and this is something we must pay attention to. Our worldwide toxin load has skyrocketed over the past few decades, and almost everything we use in our day-to-day lives is made from synthetic chemicals. Just between the years 1970 and 1995, synthetic chemical production tripled, jumping from about 50 million tons to 150 million tons yearly. That number is much higher today. The reality is that the Environmental Protection Agency (EPA) doesn't even know how many chemicals are out there. Their inventory list has about 85,000 chemicals on it, but they don't really know exactly how many are currently used in the marketplace. Scary, right? The Toxic Substances Control Act (TSCA) is the legislation that's supposed to protect us from harm, but it's far from bulletproof. Basically, it asks the question: Does a chemical pose "an unreasonable risk" of injury to health or the environment? But what qualifies as an "unreasonable risk" is nebulous. The act doesn't say whether something is safe, and there isn't much regulatory oversight. Although the TSCA was amended in 2016, only 9 chemicals have been banned in the United States since it was put in place about forty years ago, and 60,000 chemicals created before 1976 were exempted from safety testing. That's a lot of unregulated chemicals floating around.

THE FILTHY FIVE — THE WORST IMMUNE OFFENDERS

After reading the first part of this chapter, you might be feeling discouraged, depressed, or hopeless. Admittedly, when you first start learning about toxins in the environment it can seem like toxins are so pervasive that we'll never be able to avoid them entirely—how could we? If that's how you're feeling, you are correct. The reality is that we'll never be able to avoid toxins entirely with the way modern life is set up and chemicals are regulated. But here's the catch—that's okay! Our immune systems are designed to be able to handle *some* toxic exposure without totally falling apart. Our goal is to reduce the toxic exposures that we do have control over, and to support our bodies to do the rest.

First, let's talk about the most heinous toxin offenders and where to find them so we can take steps to avoid them as much as possible:

- **PFAs:** This is a group of toxic fluorinated chemicals called per- and polyfluoroalkyl substances that have been around since the 1940s. They're used in many industries, such as personal care, food packaging, and textiles. Often called "forever chemicals" because they don't break down over time, they become a persistent problem by accumulating in the body. PFAs damage the immune system and have been shown to decrease the effectiveness of vaccines like those for tetanus and diphtheria.[10] They're also linked to cancer, hormone disruption, and low birth weight.[11] You can find PFA chemicals on coated paper and cardboard containers used to hold fast foods, and also on microwave popcorn bags. PFAs are also in PTFE, aka Teflon, and other nonstick coatings on pans and utensils. Popular brands like Scotchgard, Stainmaster, and Gore-Tex, and clothes labeled stain- or water-repellent, also usually contain PFA chemicals; and they're often found in stain-resistant fabric and carpets.

Because they're so ubiquitous and were not reported by the EPA as hazardous until 2006, the possibility of groundwater contamination is an ever-present danger. Recently the movie *Dark Waters* dramatized the legal case between plaintiffs in West Virginia and the DuPont chemical company (they had dumped the chemical PFOA from their Teflon product illegally and ended up poisoning an entire community and its livestock). PFAs are also found in tap water, since they're not treated or screened out.[12] Yikes. In fact, it's estimated that 99 percent of Americans have PFAs in their blood. Although everyone should avoid these chemicals, those with a Hyperactive or Weak Immunotype should pay special attention. You can check your community for PFA contamination using the interactive map on the Environmental Working Group website (www.ewg.org/interactive-maps/pfas_contamination/).

- **Endocrine-disrupting chemicals:** This is a large group of ubiquitous chemicals that includes bisphenol A (BPA), phthalates, and parabens. BPA is used to make polycarbonate plastic, which adds rigidity to plastic and has been used for years in food containers, water bottles, sports equipment, and many other household items. It's also used in the lining of metal food cans to keep the metal from reacting with the food. It used to be in baby bottles until it was proved to mimic estrogen and interfere with childhood sexual development. That said, BPA also interferes with the adult hormone system, and it's not banned from all plastics. Several studies link BPA to the development of autoimmune disease based on its effect on increasing Th17 cells, making it extra important for those with a Misguided Immunotype to toss the plastics![13]

Phthalates, on the other hand, make plastic more flexible and are found in lotions, shampoo, food packaging, pharmaceuticals, cosmetics, IV tubing, and flooring. Really, they're *everywhere*. Kids with increased levels of phthalates in their urine have more allergies and asthma, as do kids with PVC flooring in their homes.[14] [15] Phthalates interfere with cytokine signaling as well as antibody production, essentially weakening our ability to fight infections.[16] If that isn't enough, evidence shows that phthalates may increase the risk of lupus and possibly other autoimmune diseases.

Parabens are preservative chemicals used in a wide variety of foods, cosmetics, and personal care products to prevent the growth of bacteria and mold. Because of their estrogen-mimicking abilities, they've been associated with higher incidence of breast cancer.[17] A higher body burden of parabens also increases the risk of developing food allergies, eczema, and asthma, so they should be carefully avoided by those with a Hyperactive Immunotype.[18]

- **Organophosphate pesticides:** Organophosphates (OPs) are a group of highly toxic insecticides that also happen to be the most widely used for farming, home gardens, and indoor insect control. They're also found in flame retardants used in furniture and clothing. Seriously. Despite several having been banned for their toxic effects, about thirty-six are still available for use in the United States, and recent studies have found residues of thirteen of them on fruits and vegetables.[19] Pesticide exposure causes antibiotic resistance in bacteria, creating so-called superbugs, which are really hard to kill.[20] It's well known that long-term chronic exposure to pesticides increases the risk of cancers such as lung cancer, prostate cancer, lymphoma, and leukemia.[21] Pesticides also cause increased oxidative stress in tissues like the brain, which ramps up inflammation. The connection between Parkinson's disease and pesticide exposure is attributed to this.[22] Other immune system effects of pesticides include increased death of immune cells like B and T lymphocytes, NK cells, and macrophages.[23]

- **Heavy metals:** We all remember the tragedy of what happened in Flint, Michigan, in 2014 when high lead levels contaminated the water. Well, the truth is that we all have small exposures to multiple heavy metals through water supplies, soil, our home environment, amalgam dental fillings, and even the foods we eat. If you live in an old house with chipping paint, and you really love sushi, you may be at risk for high lead and mercury levels. Over a lifetime this can silently build up and cause disease. For example, both arsenic and lead are associated with immune suppression, increased infections, and increased risk of cancer.[24] [25] Mercury can trigger autoimmune disease by binding to cells, changing their structure, and triggering a loss of immune tolerance.[26] I inform my Misguided Immunotypes to be very cautious about toxic metal exposures through water and food.

- **Formaldehyde:** This is a toxin that's used just about everywhere. It's present in the particleboard used in furniture, laminate flooring, and kitchen cabinets. It's a volatile organic compound (VOC) that off-gases from upholstered furniture, drapes, and many household products such as glues and paints. Avoiding formaldehyde is particularly important if you're a Hyperactive Immunotype, since it's known to trigger asthma, rashes, and allergic reactions by triggering our immune cells to trend toward Th2 dominance.[27] It's also a well-known carcinogen, which means it has been labeled "cancer-causing."

As you can see, chemicals lurk in basically every nook and cranny of your home, beauty routine, water, air, and cleaning supply cabinet. But don't get discouraged. All is not lost. By focusing on the five main immune disrupters above—and especially on the chemicals that contribute directly to your specific Immunotype—you can get smarter about reducing your chemical exposure. Every little bit counts in lowering your total body burden of chemicals over our lifetime. Which brings me to....

SUPPORTING YOUR INNATE DETOXIFICATION SYSTEM

Even if we take steps toward a less toxic lifestyle by avoiding the Filthy Five chemicals, we're still constantly detoxifying all manner of chemicals, drugs, hormones, toxins, foods, and microbes twenty-four hours a day. The more toxins we have in our blood, fat, and other tissues, the more inflammation and oxidative stress we have as well. Therefore, it behooves us to support our body's ability to detox quickly and efficiently. Now, before you get scared that I'm going to ask you to do a juice cleanse, coffee enema, or water fast, know that supporting your body's innate detoxification pathway is something you can do on a daily basis with very little effort at all—zero intense "detoxes" needed.

So how do we do it? Well, we have two phases of detoxification in the liver, and each enlists numerous enzyme pathways that are genetically controlled. Phase I, also called cytochrome P450, breaks down fat-soluble toxins and initially creates more unstable free radicals in our liver. But in phase II, a process called "bio-transformation" converts the toxins unearthed in phase I to a water-soluble form so they can leave the body with waste. The bile in our gallbladder and microbes in the gut all contribute to moving these toxins out of our bodies. So while there's all sorts of dubious advice out there on "detoxing"—like the lemon cayenne detox, the green juice detox, the apple cider vinegar detox, and ionic footbaths—what you really need are the right vitamins and minerals, which work as cofactors for the enzymes involved in detoxification, to keep things rolling along at a steady pace.

Here are just some of the substances that have been shown to upregulate our initial phase I and phase II enzymes:[28]

- Curcumin (from turmeric root)
- Diindolylmethane, from cruciferous vegetables (cabbage, cauliflower, Brussels sprouts, watercress, and broccoli)
- Quercetin, from apples, onions, strawberries, apricots, and many other fruits
- Epigallocatechin gallate (EGCG), from green and black tea
- Resveratrol, from grapes and red wine
- Rosemary
- Chicory root and dandelion
- Rooibos and honeybush tea

The simple act of eating these whole foods and ingredients regularly means that you're doing a "detox" all the time.

Although whole foods are always the best sources to enhance our natural detoxification, if you have a high burden of toxins or have genetic issues (also called SNPS, or single-nucleotide polymorphisms) that negatively impact detoxification, these supplements may help:

- **NAC (N-acetyl cysteine):** This naturally occurring sulfur-containing substance derived from the amino acid cysteine is an excellent free-radical scavenger and antioxidant. It's highly active in the lung, where it works to thin mucus, making it helpful in certain lung diseases, too. It's also been found to enhance the growth and function of T cells in immune deficiency disorders like HIV and also to increase natural killer cell levels.[29] NAC is found naturally in chicken, turkey, yogurt, cheese, eggs, sunflower seeds, and legumes. It replenishes our body's supply of glutathione, which brings us to…

- **Glutathione:** Glutathione is often referred to as the "master antioxidant" for its far-reaching capabilities in antioxidant protection and its ability to bind up heavy metals and fat-loving toxins, to increase levels of other antioxidants in the body, and to prevent cell death. It's a stinky molecule, made up of sulfur and three other amino acids, and we make it constantly in our liver. People with high toxin loads deplete their glutathione quickly, and if it's not replaced, that leaves the body open to damage from free radicals. Because of its presence in the lungs, low glutathione levels have been associated with severe cases of COVID-19.[30] Several studies have recommended using glutathione and its precursor NAC as treatment for COVID-19. I recommend making sure not only that your toxic load is minimized but also that you take in the foods that keep your glutathione optimized, such as the sulfur-rich vegetables onions, garlic, and leeks, and cruciferous veggies like cabbage, kale, watercress, collards, and broccoli. For those who aren't sensitive to dairy products, a good-quality whey protein will also boost glutathione levels.

- **Chelators:** Certain foods and nutrients bind to, or "chelate," dangerous immune-harming heavy metals like mercury, cadmium, and lead. These chelators can pull out heavy metals and transport them to the kidneys or take them to the liver, where they're dumped into bile on the way out of the body with the waste in the intestines. One of the best ways to make this happen is to consume a lot of mixed soluble and insoluble fiber every day. Substances like citrus pectin, inulin, oat fiber, bran, and psyllium can all improve the removal of toxins by binding them in the GI tract.[31] The blue-green algae chlorella has been found to lower levels of toxic mercury and lead; and several studies have shown the effectiveness of activated charcoal and zeolite clay for binding toxins.[32] [33] [34]

Toxins are impossible to avoid completely, but using the natural dietary interventions covered above and adding in some liver-supporting supplements, which we'll learn about next, go a long way toward protecting your immune system, regardless of your Immunotype.

YOUR DETOXIFYING TOOLKIT

The hard truth is that there are toxins lurking around our houses and apartments that are detrimental to our immune system. That said, reducing your toxic exposure doesn't require you to spend hundreds of thousands of dollars to build a new chemical-free home and throw out everything you own, nor do you have to start washing your hair with apple cider vinegar or using beet juice as lipstick. As recently as ten years ago, going chemical-free meant making major lifestyle adaptations and sacrifices that all but put you on the outskirts of regular society. But today, there are a ton of chemical-free beauty, cleaning, and household brands that make switching to a toxin-free lifestyle *way* easier than you think.

In this chapter's Toolkit, I've included easy actions you can take to detoxify your environment that don't require a ton of money or time; in fact, you could blow through this list in a single week. I promise—you'll never look back!

1. **Filter your water:** Given the fact that most municipal water supplies don't and cannot test for all chemicals, and you can't rely on the EPA to quickly address water toxicity problems, many of us may be regularly taking in immune-damaging chemicals, residues of pharmaceutical drugs that people flush down the toilet, microbes, or lead from lead pipes just by drinking tap water. My advice is to take things into your own hands by filtering your water. But before you go out and buy just any water filter, you should know that not all filters are created equal. In fact, carbon filters—like the perennially popular Brita system—will remove most heavy metals but not a lot of other toxins. If you can swing it, I advise investing in a better counter filter, such as the Berkey filter or an under-sink reverse osmosis filter like Aquasana to remove most toxicants. If you have the budget for a whole-house filter, go for it, as you'll have purified water to drink and also to bathe in. Here are five filter options for five different budgets, from most cost-effective to most expensive:
   - ZeroWater: Less than $50 for a pitcher water filter
   - Berkey: $200 to $300 for a countertop system
   - Aquasana: $200 to $300 for an under-sink water filter system
   - Aquasana: About $700 for whole-house water filtration
2. **Start nurturing your green thumb:** When we think about the phrase "air pollution," many of us immediately conjure up images of a factory pumping out gray smoke or the car exhaust created by a traffic jam. But did you

know that indoor air quality is often much worse than outdoor air? Because modern homes are tightly sealed, we have less airflow, which keeps the airborne toxins inside. This can be frustrating to learn at first, but it also presents a huge opportunity to reduce your exposure to toxins inside your home. And believe it or not, bringing in some inexpensive plants can make a big difference in improving the air quality. Besides, houseplants are trending. In 1989, NASA published a study of the ability of plants to remove benzene, formaldehyde, trichloroethylene, ammonia, and toluene from the air. (Peace lilies, chrysanthemums, cornstalk plants, and palms scored the highest.) Another method of purifying your air is to use a HEPA air filtration system in your bedroom and the rooms you spend the most time in. These filters can capture particles down to 0.03 microns and will remove pollen, animal dander, mold spores, and dust that can trigger allergic and irritant reactions. Some HEPA air filter brands to look for are Coway, Blueair, Austin Air, and Molekule. Several models also filter out volatile organic compounds (VOCs), which are gases emitted from household items and products like paint, air fresheners, furniture, flooring, and cleaning products. They're known irritants and some, like formaldehyde, are linked to cancer. Not all air cleaners can remove these chemicals, so read the fine print. Expert tip: Make sure to choose an air cleaner that can handle the square footage of the area you're using it in, otherwise it won't be effective.

3. **Revamp your beauty routine:** This may sound negative, but we're basically sitting ducks when it comes to chemicals in our cosmetic and personal care products. Cosmetic companies can use just about any raw ingredient in their products without any safety testing or approval.

And since both men and women put a lot of beauty products on their skin, which is the most absorbent part of the body, we get a *lot* of exposure this way. Think about it: Moisturizer, shampoo, conditioner, fragrances, deodorant, and makeup are all things we use almost every day. On average, women use 12 personal care products containing 168 chemicals each day and men use about 6 products containing 85 different chemicals. And while not all chemicals are problematic, many are hormone disruptors or allergens or have negative impacts on your immune system. The worst part is that even though they may be doing damage to your body, they're totally legal!

I've already discussed some of the commonly used chemicals in personal care—parabens, phthalates, and derivatives of formaldehyde. Studies have shown that many of these chemicals weaken the immune activity of macrophages, neutrophils, and natural killer cells, interfering with the production of cytokines used to fight infections. This can result in increased allergies, inflammation, and autoimmune issues. As I said earlier, revamping your beauty routine isn't as hard as you think. There has been an explosion in the "green beauty" industry, and there's a price point for everyone. One great option is to go to the Environmental Working Group's Skin Deep database and look up the products you currently use. This database ranks products from 1 to 10 on how safe they are; that way, you can get an idea of where you're starting from. Then use the database to find healthier alternatives or do some research online. These days, a simple Google search for "clean beauty brands" will yield hundreds of results! Many larger stores also have sections for cleaner beauty products; for example, Sephora has a "Clean at

Sephora" seal on the products that meet their safety standards, and Target also has great nontoxic, vegan, and cruelty-free options, so you don't have to spend a ton of money. There are so many safe quality products out there, so there's a lot to choose from. Some of the brands I love are:

○ ILIA for makeup and skin care
○ SheaMoisture for hair care, skin care, body care
○ Burt's Bees for skin care and body care
○ Olaplex for hair care
○ Briogeo for hair care
○ Beautycounter for makeup
○ Vapour for makeup
○ Drunk Elephant for skin care
○ Native deodorant
○ Honest beauty for makeup and skin care
○ Olive and June nail polish
○ Weleda for skin care
○ Ursa Major for skin care

Thanks to these awesome brands, and others, going chemical-free doesn't have to mean downgrading your beauty routine or damaging your bank account! Before we end this section, a word of caution: Many beauty and cleaning brands (which we'll learn about in the following section) advertise themselves as "clean," "green," or "natural" but actually contain their fair share of harmful chemicals. And unfortunately, these chemicals are so poorly regulated that companies can get away with tricking us! Always look up the actual ingredients on the ingredients list or check the products on the Environmental Working Group's Skin Deep database.

4. **Clean up your cleaning products:** Along with our personal care products, we have an arsenal of immune–damaging

chemicals under our kitchen sink. Every time we clean, we breathe in and touch substances that contribute to the total burden on our body. What kind of substances, you ask? First of all, just moving around household dust can lead to a huge exposure over time, as dust has been shown to contain phthalates, flame retardants, and other chemicals that we then inhale. So, instead of using a broom, I recommend using a HEPA vacuum cleaner, damp cloths, and mops or microfiber cloths to remove surface dust and keep it from recirculating. In addition, remove your shoes when you enter your house, which, while also being very zen, will cut down on tracking in any lawn chemicals, dirt, and other toxins. Next, purge your broom closets of any products containing chlorine bleach, ammonia, and synthetic fragrances and dyes, along with any antibacterial cleansers.

Say No to Antibacterial Soap

It may seem strange, especially considering the COVID-19 pandemic, that I'm recommending you avoid antibacterial cleansers. After all, isn't the goal to kill germs when you wash your hands? It is! But study after study has shown that plain soap and warm water are just as effective as antibacterial cleansers. Antibacterial cleansers often contain triclosan, which has been flagged by environmental, academic, and regulatory groups (including the FDA) as a hormone disruptor that may be detrimental to human health. So what about hand sanitizer? When it comes to hand sanitizer, I recommend only using it when plain soap and water aren't available. Most viruses and bacteria will be killed by ethyl alcohol and isopropyl alcohol hand sanitizer, but it can be very drying and dehydrating to your skin.

My favorite brands of cleaner include:

- ○ Seventh Generation
- ○ ECOS
- ○ The Honest Company
- ○ Mrs. Meyer's Clean Day cleaning products
- ○ Method cleaning products
- ○ Grove Collaborative

Look for labels on safe cleaning products like "MADE SAFE" and the EPA's "Safer Choice." The EWG also has their list of safe cleaning products in the Guide to Healthy Cleaning.

The bottom line is that we live in a toxic world, and our immune system gets damaged every day by the plethora of chemicals that we inhale, swallow, and touch. Copious data shows that our exposure to these toxins advances inflammation, triggers allergies and autoimmune disease, and weakens our immunity, leading to cancer and weakened immune states. The first move toward restoring your immune integrity is to decrease your exposure using the steps described above. The good news is that reducing your toxic exposure is not as difficult as it sounds! I recommend taking a weekend to create a low-toxin home. Treat your immune system by purging your house of nasty chemicals and replacing them with products that are safe and health-promoting. While you're at it, order yourself a new water filter and air purifier! Your future health will thank you.

CHAPTER 9

Nutrition—Feeding Your Immune System

If there's one thing I've learned from years of studying nutrition, it's that food is not just fuel for our bodies—it's also information. Whether we pick up a carrot, an apple, a chicken wing, or a piece of chocolate cake, we're sending a signal to our cells that they have to interpret and adapt to. This applies not just to our fat cells and muscle cells but also to the cells in our immune system, which affects how our immune system functions in fighting off infections and fending off disease.

Most of us don't really think about the messages we're sending our immune system when we eat. Admittedly, most health and wellness books centered on foods are focused on the pros and cons of specific diets like low-carb, low-fat, vegan, paleo, or other eating styles with the main goal of weight loss. Even the ones that do focus on reversing specific health issues tend to praise one single approach to eating, with not a lot of room for flexibility or personalization. This book is not that. Because when it comes down to it, as long as you're feeding your immune system a varied whole-foods diet with sources of all the macronutrients and micronutrients you need, you're going to look and feel good, too.

There are people all over the world with wildly different diets who do just great in the immune department. So, instead of getting lost in the nitty-gritty of whether you personally should eat or avoid red meat, lectins, gluten, grains, carbs, or saturated fat—the list could go on and on—this chapter is going to focus on the foods that support your immune system the best and the ones that sabotage it the most. There are, after all, some foods that are universally bad for immune health—*cough, cough,* sugar and hydrogenated oils—and others that are universally good. In fact, you've probably heard of famous immune-boosting nutrients like vitamin C, zinc, and turmeric. In this chapter, I'll dive into the science on these wildly popular supplements and tell you whether or not I think they're worth the hype. Finally, we'll look at some patterns of eating that can give you a leg up in the immune department, such as intermittent fasting to increase autophagy and supercharge immune cell health. By the end of this chapter, you'll be an expert at eating for better immune health and be able to sidestep the endless nutrition debates.

SUGAR — YOUR IMMUNE SYSTEM'S NUMBER ONE ENEMY

When the first wave of COVID-19 hit the United States in the spring of 2020, it became clear that the majority of patients dying, being placed on ventilators, and going into cytokine storms had several underlying health conditions. Among those were metabolic disorders like obesity and diabetes. As I described earlier in the book, obesity and diabetes have been surging in the United

States over the past few years, and in the case of diabetes, many people are walking around unaware that they even have it. But the real question that had many people puzzled at the beginning of the pandemic was: *Why does diabetes make it harder to fight a respiratory virus?* Well, first of all, we know that the SARS-CoV-2 virus can actually make blood sugar control worse in the short term. It does this by binding to the ACE2 receptors found on the beta cells of the pancreas, which produce insulin, and can potentially throw people with diabetes into a very dangerous blood sugar state.[1] In addition, having diabetes itself means that you're in a chronic low-grade inflammatory state, which taxes the body's innate immune system and makes it slower to jump on pathogens when they enter the body. So when COVID-19 inevitably overwhelms the innate immune system cells, the T cells of the adaptive immune response make a last-ditch Hail Mary pass to protect the body by spewing out inflammatory cytokines like IL-6, IFN-γ, and TNF-α. This is often the cause of overwhelming sepsis, respiratory distress, clotting, and death caused by COVID-19.

You might be wondering why I'm telling you all this. Well, it's part of my not-so-secret plan to convince you that when it comes to the immune system, your diet *really matters*. And when it comes to nutrition, no ingredient is more detrimental to your immune health than sugar. When you have high blood sugar—which is caused by many factors, but the biggest is consuming too much sugar in your diet—it starts a vicious cycle of insulin resistance and obesity that drives up inflammatory cytokines, damages blood vessels, and activates the immune system to repair those areas. This creates a major distraction for the immune system, and basically paves the way for dangerous bacteria and viruses—like COVID-19—to slip through our body's defenses.

That might all seem like very bad news, especially if you've already been diagnosed with prediabetes or diabetes. But it's not.

Why? Because type 2 diabetes doesn't have to be permanent. Eliminating excess sugar from your diet can not only end this vicious cycle, it can reverse it completely. Becoming more metabolically healthy through dialing back your sugar consumption is one of the most effective ways to improve your immune system, regardless of your primary and even secondary Immunotype. You may be thinking "I'm not really a sweets person, I don't need to worry about this!" but even if you don't eat donuts, candy, soda, cakes, or cookies regularly, having too many simple carbs like bread, pasta, rice, potatoes, granola, or even certain fruits and juices may be silently driving up your blood sugar without your knowledge. Sugar is hiding everywhere—it's in ketchup, salad dressings, and coffee drinks as well as juice, yogurt, cereal, and protein bars. It's even in supplements—check your gummy vitamins! I'm all about preventive care, especially when it comes to an insidious disease like diabetes, and recommend that the first step you take in your nutrition journey—regardless of your age—is to ask your doctor to perform a fasting hemoglobin A1c and a fasting insulin test even if your fasting blood glucose is normal. Hemoglobin A1c measures your average blood sugar over the previous three months, so even though your blood sugar may be normal the day you see your doctor, the reality may be otherwise. There are even at-home tests now, so you can test yourself!

Once you've got an idea of where you stand on the blood sugar spectrum, you can take the steps below for better health. The good news is that by following my advice in Chapters 5, 6, and 7, you're already taking big steps toward healthier blood sugar. Why? Because studies have shown that just one poor night of sleep can negatively affect blood sugar levels, your stress hormone cortisol causes spikes in blood sugar in the short and long term, unhealthy gut bacteria can literally cause you to crave sugar (it's true, look it up!), and a lack of exercise is one of the biggest contributors to diabetes.[2] Taking healthy steps in any of these areas will help protect your blood sugar health—but this chapter is about nutrition, so now I'll give you my Blood Sugar Health Mini-Toolkit:

- **Remember that sugar is addictive:** Have you ever heard someone say that sugar is as addictive as cocaine and thought they were exaggerating? Well, they weren't. Sugar activates our opiate receptors, the same areas of the brain as the world's most addictive and life-ruining drugs. Even worse, sugar is all around us and completely legal and unregulated. Kicking a sugar habit is no easy feat! It's important to remember this as you get started so you don't feel defeated. My advice is to start by eliminating sugars little by little to ensure your success. It's hard to go cold turkey, as quitting sugar can cause a withdrawal effect in the brain that triggers cravings, irritability, and fatigue. In addition, if you're used to propping yourself up with a sugary coffee or a cookie in the afternoon or even just eating fruity yogurts and granola in the morning, your blood sugar is going to go through some ups and downs the first few days or even weeks before you feel good. But push on through. It's so worth it, as, in addition to helping your immune health, your energy levels will stabilize, your skin will become clearer, and you'll lose weight! Start slowly on the following guidelines by making small reductions in sugar every few days and celebrating your wins.
- **Cut back on obvious sugars:** This means candy, soda, cake, and, yes, the sugar-bomb Starbucks drinks many of us love so much. These foods don't provide any nutritional value and contain massive amounts of sugar. Instead, opt for dark chocolate, berries, or another low-sugar treat so you don't have to remove desserts or sweet treats completely.

You don't have to take out all sugary foods forever. The occasional dessert is okay! But at the beginning it's important to get to a place where your blood sugar is stable and healthy, so it's important that you kick those foods to the curb.

- **Check every label:** Once you've cut back on obvious sources of sugar in your life, it's time to check the amount of added sugar in every item in your pantry. When I mentioned earlier that sugar is hiding everywhere, I wasn't exaggerating. Check everything—even items that are advertised as "low in sugar" or "healthy." The average American takes in about 17 teaspoons, or 71 grams, of added sugar a day, but the American Heart Association recommends no more than 6 teaspoons, or 25 grams, of added sugar a day for women and 9 teaspoons of sugar, or 36 grams, daily for men.[3] This would be a great starting point for most people, but I would advocate that you aim even lower if you can. Remember, we still get natural sugars from fruits, vegetables, and grains as well, so we're certainly not deficient! Added sugar has many names, such as sucrose, high-fructose corn syrup, molasses, barley malt, agave, maple syrup, caramel, and honey, to mention a few.

- **Eat more fiber:** If sugar is poison, fiber is the antidote. Fiber not only keeps your digestion regular, it also helps slow the absorption of sugar into your bloodstream, which protects you from blood sugar spikes. Lack of fiber is another reason why sodas, fruit juices, and sugared coffee drinks are so detrimental to your health—they contain a ton of sugar and none of the blood-sugar-protecting fiber that fresh whole plant-based foods have. Your best sources of fiber are vegetables, fruits, whole grains, legumes (not flours), and nuts and seeds. Both soluble fiber (which dissolves in the colon) and insoluble fiber (which does not) are necessary for maintaining blood sugar in a healthy range and keeping our gut microbes fed. Some of my favorite high-fiber foods are black beans and lentils, steel-cut oats, avocados, buckwheat, Brussels sprouts, pears, raspberries, barley, and flaxseed. If you feel that you can't get enough fiber in your diet, try adding whole psyllium husk, hemp seeds, or chia seeds on top of soups and salads and in smoothies.

- **Nutrients over calories:** One way to help yourself get off the roller coaster of blood sugar is to concentrate on adding more nutrient-dense foods to your diet, with lots of protein and healthy fats, instead of worrying so much about calories. You don't need to go low-carb, just choose the "right" carbs—in fact, eating carbs in the form of vegetables, beans, whole fruits, and nuts and seeds is a great way to keep those hunger pangs at bay while also delivering mineral- and vitamin-rich foods that will prevent you from hankering for that late-afternoon cupcake or late-night ice cream. Track your food intake for about five days on a free app like MyFitnessPal or Cronometer. No judgment, just log it honestly to get a snapshot of where you are. Then look to see how much added sugar, fiber, and other nutrients you're actually getting. Try it! This is something I have all my patients do. It's eye-opening and really allows you to see where your starting point is.

So now that you understand how sugar creates metabolic disorders, blood sugar imbalance, and immune system dysfunction, let's move on to a more positive note and talk about the amazing ingredients nature provides that actually support immune health.

THE POWER OF POLYPHENOLS

You may have heard the advice to "eat the rainbow," meaning to consume a diet filled with brightly colored fruits and veggies. But do you know exactly why that is? It's because these colorful foods are chock-full of polyphenols, the chemicals that create the beautiful pigments in fruits and veggies. These incredible plant chemicals are produced by plants to defend themselves against outside stressors like radiation, bacteria, viruses, and parasites. Amazingly, when we eat them, we reap these benefits too. Anything that's naturally going to give us extra protection from outside threats is great for our immunity. Therefore, in an effort to keep it simple and avoid all the endless debates about nutrition in the wellness world, I'm going to focus on what's good for all of us and our immunity: boatloads of polyphenols.

One of the main benefits of polyphenols is that they act as antioxidants, which fight free radicals in the body and prevent oxidative stress and cellular damage. Even if you're doing all you can to live a healthy lifestyle, we all deal with free-radical exposure from our surroundings every day. Free-radical damage comes from toxins, chronic stress, ultraviolet light, substances like alcohol and tobacco, and chemicals in the air, water, and food. We even generate free radicals as a by-product when our own cells create energy from the food we eat. Free radicals do their damage to our tissues by inciting an immune inflammatory response. Because of this, we need a constant stream of free-radical scavengers, which, luckily, we can get from the antioxidants in food.

There are many, many polyphenols in the food we eat, but I recommend focusing on a few because they're multitalented when it comes to upgrading our immune balance. I'll talk about some of these in more depth in Chapter 10 when I discuss

Immunotype-specific supplements. One of the most powerful polyphenols is epigallocatechin gallate (EGCG), found in high amounts in green tea. EGCG can improve microbiome balance, help reduce free-radical damage to skin from UV light, and reduce cataracts and glaucoma.[4] [5] Studies also show that it can modulate the creation of TH1 and Th17 cells, reducing the risk of autoimmunity.[6] So that cup of matcha can be very good for a Misguided Immunotype. Resveratrol, the polyphenol famous for supposedly making red wine a "health food," is found naturally in berries and grapes; recent studies show that resveratrol helps with obesity and blood sugar regulation by inducing changes in the gut microbiota.[7] It's also associated with improving longevity and reducing chronic inflammation. Another heavy-hitter is quercetin. Quercetin is abundant in fruits and veggies, but especially in onions and apples. (Hence the saying "An apple a day keeps the doctor away.") Quercetin also helps keep the gut healthy by improving microbe diversity in the gut, reduces inflammation, and improves allergy symptoms.[8] [9]

More on supplements in Chapter 10, but for now, know that the best immune-supporting nutrition advice I can give you — regardless of your Immunotype — is to eat a diet rich in polyphenols. A quick internet search will yield a lengthy list of the most polyphenol-rich foods to incorporate into your diet, but here are my top ten:

1. Berries, such as blueberries, strawberries, blackberries, and raspberries
2. Artichokes, spinach, chicory, and red onions
3. Red and green grapes
4. Olives and olive oil
5. Coffee and black and green tea
6. Hazelnuts, pecans, and almonds

7. Apples, black currants, and cherries
8. Flaxseeds, freshly ground
9. Dark chocolate with at least 75 percent cacao
10. Spices such as cloves, peppermint, and star anise

All of these foods are easy to incorporate into your everyday routine and will pack a serious punch of antioxidants to help you bring balance to your immune system and reduce free-radical damage and inflammation. If you want to see how your favorite foods stack up on the polyphenol scale, check out the polyphenol explorer database at phenol-explorer.eu/foods.

Cutting down on sugar and increasing your intake of polyphenols are the foundation of an immune-friendly nutrition program, but it would be impossible to write this chapter without mentioning famous immune-protective nutrients like vitamin C, vitamin D, and zinc. We've all heard of these—they're touted as immune saviors in pharmacies, in health food stores, and in every nook and cranny of the internet. But is there truth to all the hype? Keep reading to find out.

IMMUNE SYSTEM SUPERSTAR VITAMINS AND MINERALS

Once you're covering your bases with brightly pigmented polyphenol-rich foods, you can also benefit from bumping up your intake of foods chock-full of immune-specific nutrients, especially if you're dealing with an acute infection or just trying not to get sick. In some cases, larger doses of these nutrients in the form of supplements can really improve your immune health as well. What I'll say before we get into specifics is that it's important to exercise caution when it comes to supplements, especially those that are marketed heavily and currently trendy. That's not to say that supplements can't be helpful—I suggest supplements to my patients all the time—but supplements cannot replace a wholesome, nutrient-dense diet.

This is where tracking your nutrition intake for a few days can tell you whether you really do get enough essential vitamins and minerals—such as zinc or vitamin C—on a daily basis. If you aren't getting enough, you can follow my recommended dosages for supplementation. Even better, you can work with an integrative or functional medicine practitioner to establish a tailored, personalized supplement routine that will bring you benefits. Oftentimes when you just take "what everybody else is taking," you can end up taking low-quality supplements, the wrong dose, or the wrong form of the nutrient and not getting the benefits you're looking for. I see this happen all the time—and it gives supplements a bad reputation. So, before you empty your bank account buying all the immune supplements in your Instagram feed and then find yourself with a supplement graveyard in your medicine cabinet a few months later, read up on the nutrient and decide whether you really need it. Supplements are an unregulated industry, and the highest-quality products, which use the best raw material, employ third-party oversight, and contain what they say they contain, tend to be more expensive. One of my favorite resources for consumers is ConsumerLab.com (https://www.consumerlab.com), which independently tests many supplements for purity and potency.

Now that that's out of the way, let's jump into the immune system superstars. These are nutrients that all Immunotypes should maximize in their diets. Let's start with the most famous of them all—vitamin C.

Vitamin C (Ascorbic Acid)

Just about everyone knows that vitamin C is important for your immune system, and you've likely been told to take it when you're feeling run-down, are traveling, or have a cold. Vitamin C is, admittedly, integral for a strong innate and adaptive immune system. It accumulates in neutrophils and not only makes them powerful killers of microbes, but also helps prevent chronic inflammation afterward when your cells are cleaning up the mess. Vitamin C also improves skin integrity, which is a powerful barrier to infection, prevents sun damage by sopping up free radicals, improves wound healing, and promotes collagen production. (That's why you see it in so many face serums these days.)

We can't make vitamin C on our own, and we don't store it in our bodies, either, so we need to constantly get it from food. And although we don't see many overt vitamin C deficiency diseases like we did in the past when scurvy was common, we do see them, especially in smokers and regular alcohol drinkers. Vitamin C deficiency has consequences aplenty; it has been linked to a higher risk of heart disease, diabetes, cancer, and sepsis.[10] Intravenous vitamin C has even shown up on COVID-19 treatment protocols around the world. This is because it may attenuate the cytokine storm that can occur in late-stage COVID-19, which often leads to organ failure, clotting, and death.[11] One meta-analysis of vitamin C in ICU patients with COVID-19 showed that high-dose vitamin C decreased both time on a ventilator and length of stay by 8 percent, and large-scale trials are ongoing to learn more.[12] Multiple studies associate low vitamin C levels with increased incidence of colds and flu in the elderly. Vitamin C also seems to shorten the duration of a cold and lessen the chest pain, chills, and fever that accompany respiratory infections.[13] In addition, vitamin C is cheap, with almost no side effects, save a little diarrhea if you take too much, so really it's a win-win.

However, before you reach for a supplement, remember that the best way to cover your nutrition bases is through real, whole foods. The top vitamin C–rich foods to add to your diet are:

- Red and green peppers
- Acerola cherries
- Oranges
- Lemons
- Guava
- Black currants
- Grapefruit
- Kiwis
- Strawberries
- Broccoli
- Kale
- Brussels sprouts

Overall, vitamin C is famous for immune health for a reason. It's incredibly important and can shorten the duration of infection as well as help your body recover from the inflammation caused by your immune response. Because of this, I often recommend vitamin C supplements to my patients, especially those with a Weak or Smoldering Immunotype. A good dose to start with is 500 mg twice daily for maximum absorption.

Vitamin E

This fat-soluble vitamin is actually a group of about eight different substances called tocopherols and tocotrienols that are found naturally in foods like nuts, seeds, and their oils. Because we store vitamin E in our fat and cell membranes, we don't have to get it every single day like vitamin C. But we still need regular doses, because it plays the most important role in protecting our cells from free-radical damage. In fact, one of the biggest triggers of heart disease is free-radical-damaged cholesterol, aka oxidized LDL—something that vitamin E may prevent. Vitamin E also has anticancer properties and may protect against cataracts and Alzheimer's disease as well.[14] Vitamin E–deficient moms are more likely to have children with asthma, and a study of kids with asthma showed that they were more likely to be vitamin E deficient than nonasthmatics.[15] Vitamin E can also be helpful for short-term, acute upper-respiratory illness. For example, nursing home residents who took 200 mg of vitamin E daily for a year had fewer colds, probably because vitamin E can increase the infection-fighting Th1 cytokines like IFN-γ, which declines with age.[16] Good sources of vitamin E include:

- Sunflower seeds
- Wheat germ oil
- Almonds
- Hazelnuts
- Peanuts
- Avocados
- Trout
- Salmon
- Spinach
- Swiss chard

Clearly, vitamin E has many benefits, and I often recommend it to my patients, especially if they have a cardiovascular-related chronic disease or are over fifty and suffering from a Weak

Immunotype. Stick to a supplement containing 200 to 400 IU of mixed tocopherols daily, and remember to take it with a meal containing some fat for better absorption.

Carotenoids and Vitamin A

Carotenoids are a group of plant chemicals that are potent anti-inflammatories and antioxidants. Some of the most common carotenoids come from colorful vegetables and fruits, such as lycopene, found in tomatoes, and lutein and zeaxanthin, found in dark leafy greens. However, the carotenoid beta-carotene is the precursor to vitamin A (also known as retinol or retinoic acid), and it's also what makes our carrots orange and squashes yellow. Beta-carotene converts to vitamin A in the intestinal tract, and it's an immune system powerhouse. In fact, the biochemist Dr. Bruce Ames includes carotenoids in his list of longevity vitamins because of their ability to optimize health. Studies have shown that low levels of carotenoids in the diet have been associated with a myriad of diseases, including multiple cancers, macular degeneration, metabolic disease, and cardiovascular diseases, as well as inflammation and immune dysfunction.[17]

Both beta-carotene and vitamin A are crucial for maintaining healthy vision and keeping skin barriers intact and functioning. In fact, Retin-A, the bestselling antiwrinkle cream, is basically derived from vitamin A. The ability to maintain a robust skin barrier, GI tract, sinuses, and lungs helps our first line of immune defense.[18] Vitamin A can also boost antibody production from B cells and lower inflammation in asthmatic lungs.[19] It's a key player in improving autoimmunity because it increases calming regulatory T cells, which oppose the inflammatory Th17 cells responsible for most autoimmune disease.[20] Vitamin A also works in the gut to encourage tolerance to foods, thereby reducing food allergies.[21]

So basically, it's a jack-of-all-trades nutrient. You can find vitamin A and carotenoids naturally in foods like:

- Carrots
- Squash
- Tomatoes
- Asparagus
- Beef liver
- Beets
- Mustard and collard greens
- Grapefruit
- Mangoes
- Watermelon
- Egg yolks
- Turkey

As you can probably guess, vitamin A is a critical nutrient for all four Immunotypes. It has been shown to help ward off infections, prevent chronic disease, decrease chronic inflammation, and even quell a hyperactive or confused immune system. The good news is that even though only a few are listed above, carotenoids are found in virtually every plant-based food—so load up your plate with colorful fruits and vegetables to get your daily dose of vitamin A.

One caveat: Because of genetic variability, up to 45 percent of individuals don't convert beta-carotene readily to vitamin A, which is the case with me.[22] You can find this out through genetic testing or by just testing your vitamin A levels. Preformed vitamin A only comes from animal foods like liver, eggs, chicken, and beef. You can also get it from supplementing with cod liver oil. This is a problem if you're vegan, so supplementing with synthetic vitamin A may be your best bet. I talk more about specific needs for vitamin A in Chapter 10, but you should limit your supplemental vitamin A to 10,000 IU or less daily and take it with food.

Vitamin D

Although not technically an antioxidant, vitamin D is arguably the most important immune-modulating nutrient that exists. We call it a vitamin, but it's actually a hormone with a structure similar to cholesterol and sex hormones. Although we can produce vitamin D in the body through interactions with sunlight, data from 2020 shows that 35 percent of American adults and 60 percent of US elderly are vitamin D deficient.[23] This risk increases if you're obese, smoke, or live in a nursing home. The list of benefits of vitamin D to your immune system is extensive, and the crazy thing is that most primary doctors rarely check it. In fact, it's not even a recommended screening test, even though several large-scale studies have shown that adequate vitamin D levels decrease your chance of dying from multiple diseases.[24] It's also important to know that the range used in most commercial labs is so wide that you'll likely be told that your vitamin D levels are "fine" even if they're barely sufficient. In my practice, I consider "optimal" vitamin D levels to be between 50 and 80 ng/mL, but anything over 30 ng/mL is considered "fine" in conventional medicine. It seems, however, that the medical community is finally waking up to the importance of vitamin D. Vitamin D is a true immune modulator. In fact, all of your immune cells have receptors for vitamin D, so regardless of immunotype, it can strengthen, calm, and balance your immune system. Here are just some of the benefits of this incredible hormone:

- Vitamin D balances our T1 and Th2 cells; and, like vitamin A, it induces more regulatory T cells and lowers Th17 cell numbers, directly discouraging autoimmunity.[25] [26] Low vitamin D has long been linked with higher instances of autoimmune disease, in particular multiple sclerosis, which also has greater prevalence in higher-latitude areas of the world where there's less sun.[27]

- Vitamin D makes our innate immune system more active and efficient at killing bacteria and viruses. In fact, studies have shown that vitamin D reduces the frequency and severity of upper-respiratory-tract infections.[28] Back in the day when tuberculosis was a disease without a cure, patients were sent to sanitariums, where they would sit out in the sun, which likely helped them because of increased vitamin D levels.

- Recent studies show that COVID-19 patients have worse outcomes, including cytokine storms, if they're vitamin D depleted. Researchers are advocating for vitamin D to be included in treatment regimens to prevent and treat severe COVID-19.

The take-home here is that vitamin D deserves all the attention it gets—and it sure does get a lot of attention! Unfortunately, getting adequate vitamin D isn't as easy as eating colorful fruits and veggies. Vitamin D isn't found in that many common foods. It's found naturally in fatty fish like tuna, mackerel, and salmon; and some dairy products and soy milks are fortified with vitamin D. The best way to get vitamin D is to get at least twenty minutes of direct sunlight on your bare skin every day. Unfortunately, if you're like me—a Northeasterner who doesn't like the cold— that just isn't in the cards during the winter. Because of this, I recommend that almost everyone supplement with vitamin D during the winter months and that you test your vitamin D levels each year to see where they fall. Recommended doses depend on what your levels are, but starting with 2,000 IU, taken with food, is a safe bet, and then you can titrate up as needed.

Selenium

Selenium is a relatively unknown mineral but a powerhouse antioxidant. It halts inflammation by being a free-radical scavenger and can strengthen antibody immune defenses as well as immune responses to viruses and tumors. Optimizing selenium levels may lower your risk of several types of cancer, such as prostate and colorectal cancer.[29] It's also helpful in diverting autoimmune disease and can lower antithyroid antibodies in Hashimoto's thyroiditis.[30] Selenium is an antiaging mineral and seems to slow down the immune senescence that occurs with aging.[31]

So where do you find this amazing antioxidant? The richest source of selenium in food is Brazil nuts—amazingly, eating just two Brazil nuts every day gives you all the selenium you need! Other sources are seafood, organ meats, and some grains. Selenium levels in foods vary widely because it all depends on the selenium level in the soil, which means you may need to supplement. If you eat a strictly vegan diet and don't like Brazil nuts, I'd consider supplementing with about 200 mcg of selenium daily. Selenium doesn't get the same attention as vitamin D or C, but it's a critical piece of the healthy immune system puzzle nonetheless.

Zinc

If you peruse the aisles of your local drugstore looking for something to help your cold and flu symptoms, you'll likely see many products containing zinc. Why? Because zinc has far-reaching positive effects on the immune system. Zinc is the second-most-abundant trace mineral in the body after iron, but according to the World Health Organization (WHO), at least one-third of the world has a zinc deficiency.[32] Zinc is a crucial micronutrient, as it regulates development of both our innate and adaptive immune systems.[33] For example, T and B cells don't grow as well without adequate zinc, NK cells and macrophages kill much less effectively, and cytokine production is sluggish. Zinc also protects membranes from being attacked by free radicals, so it can counter the inflammation from day-to-day living and help with cleanup after attack by a pathogen.

The recommendation based on the data from thirteen studies is to supplement with zinc at the earliest sign of common cold symptoms in order to shorten the cold's duration.[34] Besides hindering the common cold, zinc has been found helpful in HIV and in one study decreased immune failure by HIV fourfold after supplementation for just eighteen months. Many medical experts have recommended supplementing with zinc in the fight against SARS-CoV-2. Zinc is especially crucial in defending against viruses in people with risk factors like obesity, kidney disease, and hypertension, as well as the elderly, whose immune systems are weakening.

How do you ramp up your intake of zinc? The food with the highest amount of zinc just happens to be one of my favorites—oysters! Oysters have more than ten times the amount of zinc that any other food has. However, if you don't love these slimy creatures, other options are beef, crab, and lobster, as well as plant sources like pumpkin seeds, chickpeas, and cashews. It should be noted that vegan and vegetarian diets can be very low in zinc unless you're adding in especially zinc-rich foods. For that reason, I recommend zinc supplementation of 15 to 30 mg daily, especially if you have *any* immune dysfunction, have underlying diseases, are elderly, or eat a 100-percent-plant-based diet. I supplement during the fall and winter months for the antiviral and immune-bolstering effects. The good news is that besides possible short-term side effects like a metallic taste in your mouth and nausea, zinc supplements are safe and beneficial for all Immunotypes.

IMMUNE HEALTH SUPERFOODS

It seems like every few weeks there's an article online proclaiming a new immune-boosting superfood on the scene. Well, I'm here to tell you that any nutrient-dense food that's rich in vitamins and minerals *is* an immune superfood. That said, some foods seem to stand out from the rest for their beneficial properties, and I cover them here.

Find Your Fungi

Mushrooms have been a staple in traditional Chinese medicine for thousands of years for many reasons, including their immune-balancing capabilities. And now we have modern science to explain the effects of these amazing fungi, which, depending on the species, can boost, redirect, or modulate our immune activity. Several mushrooms in particular can help our immune system health. I'm going to start with my personal favorite: maitake (also known as hen-of-the-woods or chicken-of-the-woods). These are my favorite not only because they make delicious tacos, but also because they're rich in beta-glucans. Beta-glucans increase the activity of phagocytic cells like neutrophils, as well as stimulating NK cells to be better cancer hunters.[35] Maitake seem to be more immune-stimulatory, as they increase Th1 cytokines, so they're a great option when trying to fight bacterial and viral infections or if you have a Weak Immunotype.

Shiitake mushrooms are another favorite of mine. They're

commonly used in Asian cooking and have been found to have immune-stimulating activities. Studies show a pattern of immune-boosting benefits, such as an increase in natural killer cell and killer T cell activity—both advantageous in conquering viruses and cancer cells.[36] At the same time, shiitake extracts have also been found in the lab to protect human lung cells against the ravages of out-of-control cytokine storms.[37]

Unfortunately, not all immune-boosting fungi are palatable enough to end up in a taco, which is why you often see them in supplement form. One example of this that you might find on the hiking trail is *Coriolus versicolor,* also known as turkey tail. (That's because—you guessed it—it looks like splayed-out turkey plumage!) In tincture and dried form, this mushroom's active components have also been shown to increase the activity of natural killer cells and cytotoxic T cells, especially in cancer.[38] *Coriolus* encourages an increase in proinflammatory cytokines and boosts the production of IgG antibodies in the face of infections.

Lastly, there's the reishi mushroom, which has also been shown in several mouse and human cancer studies to increase the Th1 cytokine response and help make chemotherapeutic drugs more effective.[39] In addition, extracts of reishi promote the immune response against certain strains of herpes virus.[40]

Mushrooms can be great for immune health, especially if you have a Weak Immunotype, but good-quality options can be expensive, so if you need to be budget-conscious, I'd recommend focusing on the less-expensive immune-balancing recommendations in this chapter.

The Magic Turmeric Root

If I had to pick one culinary compound out of nature's apothecary for its immune-supportive effects, I'd go with turmeric root. This bright yellow–orange root is not only a staple in Indian cooking but contains a pretty magical compound called curcumin. Curcumin has so many beneficial effects on your immune system that it would be impossible for me to cover them all. Here are some highlights:

- It works as a potent antioxidant and anti–inflammatory by blocking NF-κB and blocking the inflammatory cytokine TNF-α.[41]
- It has been shown to improve gut health and has shown efficacy in animal models of inflammatory bowel disease like Crohn's and ulcerative colitis.[42]
- It can buffer high cortisol levels.[43]
- It encourages the growth of beneficial strains of bacteria in the gut like *Bifidobacterium* and *Lactobacillus* species and lowers other disease-causing and pathogenic bacterial strains.[44]
- It can suppress some of the immune changes at the root of autoimmune diseases, while generally helping to reduce chronic inflammation throughout the body.[45]
- It can relieve pain as much as NSAIDs do, without the gastric side effects.[46]
- It's effective for minimizing joint swelling in rheumatoid arthritis.[47]

Turmeric is a great spice to use in cooking, although it does impart a bright yellow hue to your skin, tongue, and teeth; and, because it's not well absorbed in the GI tract, you'd need to eat gobs of it to achieve immune-modulation effects. Given that, curcumin supplements are the best way to get this beneficial compound. As you can probably guess after reading the above, pretty much everyone, regardless of Immunotype, can benefit from taking curcumin. Dosages vary based on need. For general health, I recommend about 1,000 mg a day in divided doses, to be taken with food.

Ginger

Another amazing root is the spicy, aromatic gingerroot. Similar to turmeric (the two are related), ginger has strong anti-inflammatory and antioxidant properties. Ginger contains compounds called gingerols, which show promise in preventing cardiovascular disease by reducing oxidative stress in blood vessels as well as inflammation in the area.[48] Animal studies have revealed that ginger extract, thanks to its strong antioxidant properties, may help prevent alcohol-induced liver disease and can also block the kidney damage created by chemotherapy drugs.[49] [50] In addition, ginger has amazing antibacterial properties and has been shown to kill multidrug-resistant bacteria as well as certain fungal infections.[51] [52] I use it all the time in patients who have nausea, bloating, and other GI complaints from imbalances in their microbiome.[53] You can incorporate fresh gingerroot in smoothies and many other recipes, make fresh ginger tea, or grab a bottle of ginger juice at most juice bars and cafés to drink plain or dilute in water.

Broccoli Sprouts

Everyone knows broccoli is good for you, but recently, a good deal of attention has been focused on broccoli sprouts, a potent source of one of the most immune-supportive biochemicals — sulforaphane (SFN). On its own, SFN has been shown to increase the levels of several antioxidant compounds. It accomplishes this by inducing a compound in our cells called NRF-2. This is sometimes called the "master regulator" of antioxidants, which means it helps upregulate the production of other antioxidants. NRF-2 has been shown to play a role in lowering inflammation in many diseases like cancer, chronic obstructive pulmonary disease (COPD), and liver disease.[54] Most cruciferous vegetables, such as broccoli and cauliflower, contain large amounts of a precursor chemical called glucoraphanin, which converts to sulforaphane during digestion. However, young broccoli sprouts contain between ten and a hundred times more sulforaphane than broccoli. That means that eating one ounce of broccoli sprouts can deliver between ten and a hundred times more sulforaphane than mature broccoli![55] In a trial involving forty overweight adults who ate broccoli sprouts daily for ten weeks, they had a significant reduction of inflammatory cytokine levels and C-reactive protein—a marker of chronic disease.[56] The best way to eat broccoli sprouts is raw—for instance, in salads—because sulforaphane is easily broken down by cooking. Aim to eat two ounces of broccoli sprouts a week. You can easily grow your own sprouts from seeds at home in just a few days using a Mason jar and water. If you can't get your hands on broccoli sprouts, sulforaphane is also available to take as a supplement. I recommend starting with 50 to 100 mg a day.

Garlic

Not only does garlic make everything taste more delicious, but this pungent vegetable has multiple compounds that modulate the immune system. Studies on garlic find that it's immune-stimulating, increasing the activity of macrophages, NK cells, and lymphocytes.[57] At the same time, garlic is anti-inflammatory and can be cardioprotective by lowering cholesterol and blood pressure.[58] It's also fabulous for fortifying our gut microbiota, for several reasons. It can increase levels of beneficial bacteria like *Lactobacillus;* it's known to be antibacterial, antiviral, and antifungal; and it can balance gut dysbiosis that may be driving inflammation.[59] You can incorporate garlic into almost any recipe— so use it whenever you can—and you can also find it in supplement form if you're not a fan of the taste.

YOUR NUTRITION TOOLKIT

If you've read any other health and wellness books, you might be surprised by the direction that this chapter has taken. Why didn't I give you an exact diet and list of what to eat and what to avoid, as everyone else seems to do? Well, my first answer is that no one diet is perfect for everyone—with few exceptions, I don't believe that there are foods out there that are "bad" for everyone. Anyone who tells you that they hold the secret to the perfect "eating plan" isn't being honest with you. We're all unique, with different needs based on our genetics and our Immunotype. Finding a doable and healthy diet for *you* takes time, trial and error, personalization, and patience. Sure, there's data across the board that some foods are detrimental to certain people, but they may not be for you. So, instead of driving yourself crazy trying all the trendy diets out there, if you want to focus on balancing your Immunotype, follow the recommendations below. If you get stuck and need more guidance, I suggest working with a functional dietitian or nutritionist to help you correct any nutrient deficiencies you might have, identify any food sensitivities, and nail down a specific nutrition plan that works for you.

To get started, incorporating the following tips will optimize your nutrition and your health:

1. **Eat less sugar:** As we learned earlier on, sugar = blood sugar issues, and blood sugar issues = inflammation, and inflammation = immune imbalance. Therefore, the best

nutrition advice I can give is to cut down on obvious sources of sugar in your life. For how to do that, refer to the Blood Sugar Health Mini-Toolkit on page 163.

2. **Eat more leafy greens:** Leafy greens are like nature's multivitamin. They contain a ton of beneficial vitamins and minerals, including the ones mentioned below, which are invaluable for your immune system. If you add leafy greens to at least two of your meals every day, you're taking a huge step toward better nutrition. My favorite leafy greens include:

   ○ Spinach
   ○ Arugula
   ○ Kale and baby kale
   ○ Swiss chard
   ○ Bok choy
   ○ Watercress

3. **Address nutrient deficiencies:** Your immune system just doesn't function well when you lack nutrients. You might not be aware that you're having problems in this area, but you may have low energy or get sick frequently. It's essential to shore up any vitamin or mineral deficiencies to have balanced immunity, especially if you have any of the deficiencies discussed in this chapter. If you can, work with a dietitian or health care professional and have nutritional labs done. If that's not realistic, keep a food diary for a week using an app on your phone or computer. Most nutrition apps will calculate the micronutrient content of the foods you're eating so you can go through and see what you might be missing. For example, you might notice that your diet is low in zinc or selenium, so you decide to supplement or eat more Brazil nuts. If your food journal doesn't reveal any trends or

deficiencies, taking a high-quality multivitamin is another great way to make sure you're covering most of your bases. This is especially important if you can't get tested for nutrient deficiencies. Multivitamins contain a nice blend of nutrients that can help you get some of the immune-boosting superingredients discussed in this chapter. And while a multivitamin typically doesn't have high enough levels of any one nutrient to totally correct a long-standing deficiency, it may help prevent it from getting worse.

4. **Reduce alcohol consumption:** Alcohol is a sneaky substance that can really derail your blood sugar, as well as other aspects of your health. Most alcoholic drinks contain a great deal of sugar in the form of carbohydrates, which indirectly raise blood sugar levels. The big culprits are mixed drinks, beer, and cider, while dry wine is lower in sugars, and hard alcohol has none. However, alcohol itself is a fuel. That's right, ethanol can be burned for fuel by our body and in fact has seven calories per gram. That's more than protein or carbohydrates have! What's more, alcohol will be burned for energy before fat, carbs, or protein. So when you're drinking alcohol with your meals, the alcohol is burned while the rest of the calories are stored as fat. This is just one of the ways that alcohol contributes to weight gain, blood sugar imbalance, and diabetes, which can sabotage the immune system over time. Another reason to limit your alcohol intake is the fact that it's toxic to gut microbes and disrupts gut-barrier function, resulting in leaky gut. It also affects both the innate and the adaptive immune response, weakening our defenses, which can put us at risk for infections and chronic inflammation. When alcohol is broken down, a toxic metabolite

called acetaldehyde is formed, which is harmful to all our cells and increases oxidative stress on the body, requiring more antioxidants to keep the peace. Alcohol is also known to damage macrophages and neutrophils in the lungs, leading to an increase in the risk for pneumonia. Studies have even shown that alcohol contributes to seasonal allergies; it's associated with an increase in common symptoms of asthma and hay fever, like sneezing, itching, headaches, and coughing. There are many ways to reduce your alcohol intake. I suggest:

- Trading your beer, wine, or cocktail for another refreshing drink, such as a sparkling water with fresh fruit or a squeeze of lime or an iced turmeric-ginger tea. There are many great-tasting nonalcoholic beers available now, too.

- Make plans that don't revolve around alcohol. The hardest part of reducing alcohol consumption is often the social aspect of drinking. Instead of meeting for happy hour, connect with your friends over a hike, a pottery class, or a healthy picnic in the park.

5. **Incorporate immune-boosting superfoods:** By incorporating mushrooms, turmeric, ginger, garlic, and broccoli sprouts in your diet, you can get a regular dose of super-immune-boosting nutrients. This can be done in so many ways: You can consume these items in the form of soups, teas, or curries, or even juice them or add them to smoothies. There are many green powders that you can add to water or smoothies that contain all of these ingredients.

If this chapter feels a little overwhelming, I'm here to tell you that optimizing your diet to support your immune system isn't as complicated as it might seem. You don't have to track your intake of polyphenols or vitamins or minerals every day to make sure you're getting enough of everything, nor do you have to eat ginger and turmeric and mushrooms daily. Why? If you eat a diverse diet full of colorful fruits and veggies as well as some of these ingredients, you'll be getting your fair share of polyphenols, antioxidants, and immune-supportive vitamins and minerals. The nutritional foundation for a healthy immune system is as simple as that! Beyond that, it's all about further optimizing and balancing your Immunotype, which is why, in the next chapter, I'll be going even deeper by giving you more Immunotype-specific supplement and nutrient recommendations.

Now you have a good sense of how sleep, stress, gut health, your environment, and nutrition influence your immune system. And while I've mentioned some Immunotype-specific tips and factors, all four Immunotypes will benefit from optimizing these five pillars. I hope you've already adopted one or two of the tips from the Toolkit at the end of each chapter. If not, that's okay. The next chapter is all about getting specific and creating a personalized Immune Restoration Plan based on your Immunotype and your lifestyle. You'll choose tips from each of the previous five chapters to add to your plan, as well as following Immunotype-specific recommendations. That way, your plan will be optimized to fit not just your Immunotype but also your preferences, budget, and needs.

Are you ready? Let's dive in.

CHAPTER 10

Rebalancing Your Immunotype

By now you should be an expert in how your immune system works and also the myriad ways that your lifestyle can enhance or detract from its function. I know it's a lot of information to absorb, but the key factor I want to impress upon you is that you have *so much more control over your health than you've been led to believe.* Yes, the challenges we face every day, from toxins in our environment and our food to our high-stress, work-until-you-drop culture, are massive obstacles—but they're obstacles that you can conquer with the right knowledge and guidance.

The previous five chapters were all about the biggest lifestyle factors that affect your immune system. And the truth is, sleep, stress, gut health, toxins, and nutrition affect all four Immunotypes equally. Anyone who walks into my office is going to get advice on these aspects of health, and that's why the Toolkit sections of those chapters featured many pieces of advice that were more about your schedule, priorities, budget, and personality than about your Immunotype. Following these suggestions is an important part of building a solid foundation for a healthy immune system.

Now, though, it's time to get Immunotype-specific. In this chapter, we're going to delve into particular things you can do that will help you rebalance your Immunotype on a cellular level and get your body back in sync.

YOU KNOW YOUR IMMUNOTYPE — NOW WHAT?

Once you've completed the quiz in Chapter 4, you should know what Immunotype or Immunotypes you are. We now get to go deeper into how we can use certain foods, supplements, herbs, and lifestyle hacks to nudge each Immunotype back into balance.

As you read the section for your Immunotype below, you'll first get a big-picture idea of the treatment approach we'll take for your specific type during the Immune Restoration Plan. Then I'll move into some tailored lifestyle and supplement suggestions that you can incorporate over the course of the plan. I recommend starting with just one of the recommended supplements and taking it for at least one week before you add in another. There's a common problem in the wellness world of overdoing it on supplements—in other words, taking way too many and starting them all at the same time so you don't know which one is working, if any! I always recommend a more tailored approach to supplements. This way you're introducing them to your body more mindfully, instead of just throwing everything and the kitchen sink at your body and hoping something works. As long as you feel no adverse effects, you can add up to three supplements during your Immune Restoration Plan. For the first thirty days I recommend taking those three, but continue them for at least sixty days before deciding whether or not they're helping you. Why? Because I find that most people need at least sixty days to see a significant change in their symptoms, and depending on the situation, sometimes you need as long as six months. Many people quit taking a supplement before it has a chance to take effect.

Remember, supplements are not pharmaceutical drugs—they're not designed to work in twenty minutes or even two weeks. In addition, discuss all supplements and herbal additions with your health care practitioner to make sure there won't be any interactions with any of your medications. Supplements may not be pharmaceuticals, but they can interact with medications, and you should not take supplements before surgery or other medical procedures.

FORTIFYING A WEAK IMMUNOTYPE

Let's circle back to Bill, who was always getting colds, felt fatigued, and had frequent IBS symptoms and cold sore outbreaks. If you draw on the knowledge you gained in Chapter 2, you might be able to guess that Bill has problems with the strength of both his innate and adaptive immune systems. The fact that he had low immunoglobulin A in his gut indicated that it might be easier for viruses and bacteria to invade and make him sick. He also presented with low protective antibodies after getting a vaccine, which might indicate poor communication between his T cells and his antibody-creating B cells. In addition, his lab results showed reactivated Epstein-Barr virus, and he'd had shingles, caused by the varicella-zoster virus. Most of us have these herpes viruses lying dormant in our bodies, but they're kept in check by our immune systems and only break out when our immune defenses falter. Bill likely has weaknesses in his killer T cells and his natural killer cells' ability to keep these viruses under wraps.

The Weak Immunotype is the type helped most by all the immune-"boosting" practices we hear about. If you have a Weak Immunotype, in general, you want to shore up any weaknesses in the cells of both the innate immune system and the adaptive immune system. This will significantly ramp up the initial response to viruses and bacteria, prevent outbreaks of dormant viruses, and create strong antibodies to protect you in the future.

Although all aspects of the lifestyle interventions I've reviewed so far are important to implement for all types, several are particularly important to boosting your immune power. Specifically, you want to do things that:

- Increase Th1 cells and cytokines, as they're crucial to fighting infection.
- Bolster B cell activity and production of antibodies, as well as natural killer cells.
- Improve the barrier function of the gut.

To accomplish these three things, the fundamental lifestyle pillar for a Weak Immunotype is sleep. Without sleep, your hormone production is off and your circadian rhythm gets out of sync. Getting adequate sleep and prioritizing your circadian rhythm are truly essential. Remember that melatonin is secreted in the earlier part of the night when you're asleep, and this activates a lot of disease-fighting cytokine activity, so you want to maximize your normal melatonin levels. This means, too, that removing blue light and wearing blue-light-blocking glasses at night are critical.

Besides these guidelines, nature's pharmacy has a lot to offer in the form of foods and supplements that can help build up the constitution of the Weak Immunotype. You can enhance the cells of the innate immune system such as natural killer cells and macrophages with these:

- **Melatonin:** If for some reason your sleep is off and you cannot avoid blue light at night, you can try low-dose melatonin a few hours before bed. Melatonin is especially important in older individuals who are experiencing "immunosenescence," or a weakening of the immune system due to age. *Recommended dosage: 1 to 3 mg one hour before sleep.*
- **Mushrooms:** As discussed in the last chapter, mushrooms have amazing components called beta-glucans that contain some pretty impressive immune-boosting properties. Cancer trials have shown that mushrooms can rev up the immune surveillance activity of natural killer cells as well as stimulate a Th1 response by increasing cytokines that help fight viruses and bacteria.[1] My personal favorites are shiitake and maitake, as they're delicious stir-fried, roasted, or in soups. Mushrooms also contain substantial amounts of antioxidants, vitamin D, and selenium.[2][3] For an extra boost to the immune system, you can also take them in supplement form. Reishi mushrooms, though not a culinary fungus (they're generally too tough to eat), stimulate both macrophages and NK cells to release more cytokines like IFN-γ and TNF-α to help fight viral and bacterial invaders. *Coriolus versicolor* (turkey tail mushroom) has been shown to boost white blood cell numbers overall, increase the activity of neutrophils, and ramp up antibody production from B cells. Both of these fungi can be found in powder and capsule form as well as in tea and coffee blends. *Recommended dosage: Take an immune-boosting mushroom blend for at least sixty days.*

- **Ashwagandha:** The root of this plant is best known as an adaptogenic supplement for stress, and it can help with anxiety and sleep problems, too.[4] However, it also promotes NK cell activity and upregulates Th1 activity, so it's very useful when you're run-down, have chronic stress, and keep getting sick.[5][6] *Recommended dosage: 300 to 500 mg twice daily for at least sixty days.*

- **Korean red ginseng:** This is a type of *Panax ginseng,* which is wildly popular in Korea and other Asian countries thanks to its multiple effects on the immune system. It also has strong antioxidant properties and may be liver-protective against drugs like acetaminophen.[7] Across the board, it has been shown to increase both neutrophil numbers and T and B cell numbers and activity. *Recommended dosage: 1,000 mg daily.*

- **Colostrum powder:** Colostrum is the powerful substance produced before breast milk, twenty-four to forty-eight hours after giving birth. It provides babies with immunity because it contains a full array of protective immunoglobulins, nutrients, and microbe-fighting substances. Luckily, colostrum is not restricted to newborns. Adults with a Weak Immunotype can also benefit, as the colostrum from cows and goats contains these same elements and is available in powdered form. Bovine colostrum provides IgG and IgA, which protect against microbial infection, repair leaky gut, and may help prevent upper-respiratory-tract infections.[8][9][10] Most people who are lactose-intolerant can tolerate colostrum. *Recommended dosage: 3,000 mg daily in powder or capsule form.*

- **Larch arabinogalactan:** Arabinogalactan is a carbohydrate found in many plants that we eat regularly, like carrots, radishes, and pears. However, one of the best sources is the Western larch tree. It's a great prebiotic fiber to support healthy bacteria in the gut, and when supplemented with the bacteria *Lactobacillus,* it can increase NK cell activity and help in healing IBS.[11] Trials in humans have shown that it can reduce the incidence of the common cold, so it's a great option for those with a Weak Immunotype.[12] *Recommended dosage: 1,500 mg daily in powder or capsule form.*

- **Elderberry:** This plant therapy has crossed over into the world of conventional medicine, and you can find it on the shelves of most mainstream pharmacies. Elderberry has been shown to help in the early stages of an upper-respiratory viral infection.[13] It does this by ramping up proinflammatory cytokines like IL-6 and TNF-α. It can be helpful for those with a Weak Immunotype at the onset of a cold. Prudent advice is to limit elderberry to mild upper-respiratory infections such as the common cold and to stop using it if there's any sign of fever or worsening of the condition. *Recommended dosage: 4 grams daily for prevention in syrup, capsule, or tablet form. Can be taken up to three times daily when you're acutely sick.*

COOLING OFF A SMOLDERING IMMUNOTYPE

We've dissected inflammation quite a bit so far, and I hope I've made it pretty clear that a healthy inflammatory response is a necessary and integral part of our daily lives and crucial to the success of the immune system. However, some of us get stuck in a pattern of low-level inflammation that doesn't resolve. Over time, it becomes detrimental to our health, since chronic inflammation is a major instigator in autoimmune diseases, allergies, heart disease, and other chronic disorders. The Smoldering Immunotype predominantly has inflammation and may not show signs (yet) of a Hyperactive or Misguided immune response.

We know that the major drivers of inflammation are mostly things that we have tremendous control over, and following the advice in the book so far will significantly reverse your inflammation and steer your body in the right direction. Those with a Smoldering Immunotype aren't necessarily immune-compromised, but their immune system is busy putting out day-to-day fires, so it may not always mount a robust response to a serious threat. However, over time, poor diet, lack of sleep, chronic stress, high blood sugar, and obesity will cause declines in immune cell health and activity. This is why I call it Smoldering: It may not be obvious that you have an immune imbalance until you get sick. Smoldering Immunotypes may also have a Th1 dominance, so they may not want to take anything that would push them further in that direction, which could make them even more inflamed. To that end, all our efforts are going to be focused on the following:

- Dismantling targets that create inflammation in our cells, including NF-κB, the inflammasome, and the production of inflammatory cytokines.
- Accelerating the resolution of inflammation so you don't get caught in the cycle of chronic immune activation.

If you scored high on the Smoldering Immunotype part of the quiz, your number one lifestyle intervention is to put a spotlight on your nutrition. This includes:

- Avoiding or minimizing alcohol
- Throwing sugar to the curb
- Eating a whole-food, organic diet full of antioxidant-rich fruits and vegetables

The Smoldering Immunotype needs to go the extra mile in reducing inflammation beyond just lifestyle choices—you need to focus on downplaying inflammatory pathways on a cellular level, so consider taking these supplements to achieve that goal:

- **Curcumin:** Is there anything this amazing substance can't do? In Chapter 9, I mentioned it as the main active ingredient in turmeric root. Curcumin can shut down inflammation on many levels. More than 120 human clinical trials have shown benefits for diseases ranging from Alzheimer's to diabetes, heart disease, and autoimmunity.[14] Although it's wonderful to add turmeric to your diet by grating fresh turmeric root into soups and stews or using the dried spice, it's almost impossible to get high enough doses in food to be therapeutic. If you're a Smoldering Immunotype, I highly recommend taking curcumin in supplement form. Curcumin is poorly absorbed from the GI tract, but more bioavailable forms—such as those with added black pepper—have been developed to increase absorption up to 400 percent.[15] That being said, you still want to take curcumin along with a fatty meal for the best results. *Recommended dosage: 1,000 mg twice daily.*

- **Resveratrol:** This polyphenol is another substance that's hard to get in therapeutic doses from food, including from its famous source: red wine. Once we metabolize it, we only have about 1 percent left, so supplementing is the best way to go. Resveratrol has been found to be effective in clinical trials for heart disease, type 2 diabetes, cancer, obesity, and aging.[16] In one study a group of diabetics took 1 gram a day for forty-five days and experienced improvements in blood sugar, insulin resistance, and hemoglobin A1c levels. Resveratrol also helps inhibit the production of amyloid brain plaques in Alzheimer's disease.[17] [18] Again, this is due to its antioxidant and anti-inflammatory effects, but it also seems to mimic calorie restriction, leading to a better metabolic profile and less disease.[19] One of the reasons resveratrol has been the darling of the antiaging community is that it increases a compound called SIRT1 in our cells, which improves endurance and longevity and decreases chronic disease. When looking for a resveratrol supplement, make sure it's 98 percent trans-resveratrol from Japanese knotweed. Take it with a fatty meal for best results. *Recommended dosage: Start with 500 mg and increase to 1 gram divided into two daily doses.*

- **Specialized proresolving mediators (SPMs):** As their name tells you, these help "resolve" inflammation. Remember in Chapter 3 when I talked about how infections drive a lot of neutrophils into the infected area to gobble up the microbes, but if there aren't enough macrophages to haul away the bacteria-filled neutrophils, it triggers a mad cycle of chronic inflammation? This is where specialized proresolving mediators step in. SPMs don't keep inflammation from happening in the first place, but instead block the continued recruitment of new neutrophils to the area. They also signal more macrophages to come in and clear away the debris, so they're crucial in resolving inflammation. Although your body can make SPMs from omega-3 fatty acids, it takes a while, so if you have a Smoldering Immunotype, your body might not be able to keep up with demand. The great thing is that because SPMs don't interfere with the creation of inflammation, they're not immunosuppressive. In addition, they're much safer to take than NSAIDs, steroids, and other anti-inflammatory medications. I love these particularly for pain and arthritis. *Recommended dosage: 2,000 mg daily.*

- **Berberine:** This compound is found in many different plants (like goldenseal, barberry, and Oregon grape) and is a huge player in downregulating inflammation and reducing oxidative stress in the body. It has strong antimicrobial properties and is commonly used to treat bacterial infections and overgrowth in the gut that may be driving chronic inflammation. Berberine has also been shown to increase insulin sensitivity and improve blood sugar regulation.[20] In fact, in a study pitting berberine against the common diabetes drug Metformin, berberine was equally effective in lowering fasting blood sugar, insulin, and hemoglobin A1c, while also lowering cholesterol and triglycerides.[21] So overall, this compound is amazing for Smoldering Immunotypes, especially those with metabolic syndrome, including obesity, high blood sugar, and heart disease. *Recommended dosage: 500 mg taken three times daily.*

There are dozens of other natural substances that have demonstrated tremendous anti-inflammatory and antioxidant effects, but the ingredients above are the ones that I have found to have good safety records and to attack several different mechanisms that drive inflammation.

CALMING A HYPERACTIVE IMMUNOTYPE

Unlike the Misguided Immunotype, where T cells and antibodies attack "self" tissues, the Hyperactive Immunotype overreacts to harmless things outside the body, like pollen and dust. When your immune system is working perfectly, it should be able to tell the difference between friends, foes, and innocent bystanders; it should be able to rapidly attack and destroy a dangerous virus while not launching a response to the family cat or the pollen outside. And yet so many of us have immune systems that do just that, and we're suffering from chronic allergies, eczema, and asthma in growing numbers every single day.

Why is it that our bodies seem to react to harmless things in our environment? Several different mechanisms are at play in the Hyperactive Immunotype. First and foremost, we know that helper T cells in people with environmental allergies, asthma, food allergies, chronic sinusitis, and allergic skin conditions are "stuck" in a Th2-dominant pattern. The Th2 cells and the cytokines they produce increase IgE antibodies, which directly cause an allergic reaction.[22] IgE also rallies other immune cells involved in allergies, like eosinophils, mast cells, and a chemical called histamine. To protect our bodies from these actually harmless substances, there's a lot of swelling, runny nose, mucus, coughing, and irritation. Although we don't know 100 percent why allergies developed in humans, there are ways to shift away from excessive Th2 dominance, lessening this tendency, starting with:

- Resolving infections and other triggers that keep you chronically inflamed.
- Using supplements to push the needle back toward Th1 activity while dampening Th2 activity and the cytokines that support it.

If you scored high on the Hyperactive Immunotype part of the quiz, your number one intervention is going to be taming the toxins in your life. Both indoor and outdoor toxins enhance a TH2 polarization while hindering a TH1 response. Substances like phthalates, pesticides, lead, and mercury, as well as chemicals in diesel particles and cigarette smoke, all enhance the allergic response by throwing off immune balance. By creating a "greener" home environment and following the recommendations in Chapter 8, you'll be doing a lot to quiet down a hyperactive response. In addition, the following supplements can be extremely helpful:

- **Quercetin:** You've learned that quercetin is a powerful flavonoid and antioxidant found in many fruits. It's a great addition to the Hyperactive Immunotype Toolkit for several reasons. It interferes with Th2 cytokines, which drive allergies, while also increasing the Th1 cytokine interferon IFN-γ, which may explain its immune-boosting effects. Quercetin also acts like an antihistamine, giving relief to allergy sufferers more immediately.[23] One product developed in Italy called Lertal, which contains quercetin and perilla (see below), is in clinical trials for allergic rhinoconjunctivitis. *Recommended dosage: 500 mg twice daily.*

- **Astragalus root:** This is a great choice to tip away from Th2 dominance toward Th1 response. It was found to improve airflow rates in children with asthma, and in other studies lowered allergy markers like high IgE antibodies and high eosinophils, which often accompany allergic reactions.[24] [25] *Recommended dosage: 500 to 1,000 mg daily of standardized dried root in capsule or tincture form.*

- **Perilla:** This plant in the mint family is one of the fifty most important compounds in traditional Chinese medicine. Perilla contains high levels of rosmarinic acid, which has been shown to significantly reduce allergy symptoms. A double-blind twenty-one-day trial of perilla significantly reduced symptoms like runny nose and itchy, watery eyes by blocking Th2 cytokines.[26] *Recommended dosage: 300 mg twice daily.*

- **Stinging nettle (*Urtica dioica*):** Stinging nettle is an herb whose leaves have antihistamine properties. A thirty-day study on the use of stinging nettle for allergy symptoms showed a significant decrease in symptoms, as well as a drop in eosinophil counts.[27] *Recommended dosage: 500 mg daily of freeze-dried root. Tinctures and teas can also be used.*

REDIRECTING A MISGUIDED IMMUNOTYPE

The Misguided Immunotype is the most complicated of all the types because it's almost always accompanied by another Immunotype, such as a Smoldering Immunotype. At its most basic, the Misguided Immunotype has missed the memo about not attacking their own tissue. Somewhere during development, self-reactive T cells slipped by surveillance and didn't get destroyed as they should have been. These T cells get activated and turn into Th17 cells, which are highly inflammatory and attack "self" tissue like it's a foreign threat. This damaged tissue then triggers an influx of other immune cells, starting the crazy cycle of ongoing inflammation. In addition, antibodies often form against "self" tissues that just perpetuate the process.

Many factors influence the way autoimmune diseases come about. First, genetics might make you more predisposed to an autoimmune condition, but your genes don't have to seal your fate. Things like infections, food, stress, and toxins play a huge role. Remember when we talked about epigenetics? Well, epigenetics is the study of how our environment influences our genetic expression and therefore our susceptibility to disease. To make matters even more complicated, people with a Misguided Immunotype have either an underlying Th1 or Th2 polarization, but then they almost always have an abundance of Th17 cells; and it's these Th17 cells that are responsible for the tissue destruction that occurs in diseases like rheumatoid arthritis and multiple sclerosis.

Despite this complexity, if you follow all the recommendations given so far in the Immune Restoration Plan and add in the recommendations from this chapter, you'll start to see improvements in your symptoms. I strongly recommend that you also pay attention to whether you scored really high on the Hyperactive or Smoldering Immunotype part of the quiz. If that was the case, I'd look at those recommendations and incorporate them as well.

Another issue with the Misguided Immunotype is that it can take much longer for interventions to balance the immune response. Part of the problem is that you have to simultaneously try to decrease inflammation, reduce Th17 cells, balance your Th1/Th2 cells, and reduce the level of self-directed antibodies. This can take months, but I urge you to stay the course and be patient. Positive changes will come! As you move through the recommendations, pay attention to which interventions seem to balance your Immunotype and discontinue anything that in any way seems to exacerbate your symptoms. Autoimmune issues are tricky, and we're all different. Sometimes a little trial and error is a necessary part of the process.

Let's go back to the case of my patient Rachel, who had rheumatoid arthritis, an autoimmune disease, as well as signs that she was developing an autoimmune disease in other areas of the body. She had a history of antibiotic use, overgrowth of pathogenic bacteria according to her stool test, and food sensitivities to gluten and soy, fueling her chronic inflammation. Her gut was a mess, and as we learned in Chapter 7, the gut is ground zero for establishing immune tolerance. That's why I want you to prioritize your gut health. Follow the recommendations in Chapter 9, focusing on fiber, fermented foods, and loads of antioxidants and polyphenols. And try an elimination diet, another very helpful tool that I use with all my Misguided Immunotypes.

Many foods are known to be strong autoimmune instigators and will continue to promote inflammation in the gut and elsewhere if you keep eating them. As an initial first step, I recommend a thirty-day removal of added sugar, alcohol, wheat, dairy, soy, eggs, corn, peanuts, and processed foods. This will allow the immune system ample time to become less reactive if any of these foods are an issue. After thirty days, you'll likely notice improvement in energy, mood, sleep, joint aches, headaches, intestinal problems, and other symptoms. The real enlightenment occurs, however, when you add back certain foods. If you add back only one food at a time for forty-eight hours, you'll notice a recurrence of symptoms if that food is a problem. Other stricter elimination diets, such as the autoimmune paleo diet (AIP), can also be used. This diet goes even further by removing nuts and seeds, legumes, grains, and even nightshade vegetables. Studies show that using AIP diets can improve intestinal diseases like ulcerative colitis, Hashimoto's thyroiditis—an autoimmune thyroid disease—and the autoimmune nervous system condition multiple sclerosis (MS).

Elimination Diets Aren't Forever

I know what you're thinking. "I'm so confused! If I eliminate all these foods, what *can* I eat? Is this forever?" I hear this from my patients all the time, and I get it! My stance is that an elimination diet should be used as a tool first and foremost. Why? For one, allergies, food sensitivities, and food intolerances are all different things. No one lab test can delineate all these different issues for you, or tell you which foods to eat and which ones to avoid. Only an elimination diet can give you that information. And some research shows that an elimination diet can be effective at improving autoimmune disease.[28] That said, there need to be many more clinical trials on elimination diets for autoimmune disease before you cut all common food-sensitivity foods out of your diet for the rest of your life. By removing some of these nutritious foods, like certain vegetables, nuts, seeds, and grains, you may be inadvertently eliminating many minerals and vitamins from your diet, along with gut-healing fiber. I have seen firsthand how months of strict elimination diets can cause food phobias, social isolation, anxiety, worsening microbiome health, and nutritional deficiencies. I highly recommend working with a trained functional medicine nutritionist or dietitian before embarking on an elimination diet.

Correcting a Misguided Immunotype is a little more complicated than correcting the three other Immunotypes. When it comes to supplements, you have to take a multipronged approach:

1. Dampen excessive inflammation, just as the Hyperactive and Smoldering Immunotypes have to do, by following the recommendations below.
2. Block damaging Th17 cell activity, which perpetuates tissue destruction in autoimmune disease.
3. Hit the off switch of an overexuberant immune response by increasing regulatory T cells. (Remember, these are the calming T cells that create more balance in your immune system.)

Here are some key tools for doing this:

- Start by following some of the interventions listed in the Smoldering Immunotype to squelch excess inflammation, such as taking curcumin, resveratrol, and SPMs.

- **Vitamin D:** I've talked about how Vitamin D deficiency is a risk factor in the development of autoimmune disease and inflammation, so having a robust amount of this vitamin is crucial. Vitamin D increases the number of regulatory T cells, which the Misguided Immunotype needs. I aim for a serum level of 50 to 80 nl/ml. Remember to get a baseline from your doctor and repeat it eight to ten weeks after starting supplementation. *Recommended dosage: If you don't know your level, a safe dosage to start with is 2,000 to 4,000 IU daily. If your level is less than 30 nl/ml, you may need 10,000 or more IU daily to reach these levels. Testing is key.*

- **Vitamin A:** In Chapter 9, I talked about vitamin A's role as an antioxidant, but it's superimportant for folks with a Misguided Immunotype because it ramps up those calming regulatory T cells,[29] especially in the gut, where autoimmune disease often starts. Vitamin A can also help heal food sensitivities, which drive autoimmunity and block the formation of tissue-destroying Th17 cells.[30] *Recommended dosage: 5,000 to 10,000 IU a day, taken with food.*

  Note: Very high levels of vitamin A can be toxic, so make sure that other supplements you take don't contain vitamin A. In pregnant women in particular, amounts greater than 25,000 IU a day can cause birth defects, and the World Health Organization does not recommend that pregnant women take vitamin A at all.[31] Most prenatal vitamins will only contain beta-carotene, for that reason.

- **Skullcap:** Baicalin is the active ingredient in a well-known Chinese herbal medicine called *Scutellaria baicalensis,* also known as Chinese skullcap. It's popular in the naturopathic medicine world for its antioxidant properties, but it's also effective in halting autoimmune activity because of its ability to block inflammatory cytokines like IL-6 and TNF-α.[32] It also blocks Th17 cells.[33] Studies have found it effective in treating arthritis, ulcerative colitis, and psoriasis.[34] [35] Additionally, it has a strong antiviral effect, so it's a great choice when an autoimmune disease is driven by an underlying viral infection like Epstein-Barr virus. *Recommended dosage: 500 mg taken twice a day.*

- **Glutathione:** Glutathione is arguably the most important antioxidant in the body, which is why it's often referred to as the "master antioxidant." Glutathione neutralizes extremely damaging free radicals that are formed in our cells from immune cell activity, detoxification, and even the day-to-day production of energy. Glutathione helps recycle other antioxidants, like vitamin C and vitamin E, which are also protective against oxidative stress. It preserves the function of regulatory T cells that can turn off an overexuberant immune response.[36] In animal models, glutathione was able to lower levels of rheumatoid arthritis antibodies, often used to track disease activity.[37] Because of the tissue damage that occurs in the Misguided Immunotype, glutathione is truly necessary.

    So where do you get this amazing substance? We make it in our bodies from amino acids like cysteine, glutamine, glycine, and sulfur; large amounts of these are found in cruciferous veggies like cabbage, broccoli, and kale. Almost everyone can benefit from glutathione, but the Misguided Immunotype has so much oxidative stress, tissue damage, and inflammation that I recommend upping your glutathione game. The best way to do this inexpensively is to take N-acetyl cysteine, also known as NAC. This is one of the most important precursors to glutathione and will help you keep up with demand if your stores are tapped. *Recommended NAC dosage: 600 to 1,200 mg a day.*

You can take glutathione itself, but there are some caveats. It's not well absorbed orally, and it's quite pricy. It also smells a bit like rotten eggs. That being said, it has been made into sublingual and liposomal formulations for better absorption. *Recommended glutathione dosage: 500 mg twice daily.*

- **Cordyceps sinensis:** Also known as the caterpillar fungus, *Cordyceps sinensis* is prized for its antiaging and heart-supportive effects. It also has anti-inflammatory effects and is useful for patients with autoimmune disease. It can increase the ratio of regulatory T cells to Th17. A drug called the Corbin capsule made from *Cordyceps,* given three times daily, was found to improve markers of disease severity in patients with autoimmune thyroid disease.[38] Although this drug is only available in China, synthetic *Cordyceps* is widely available. *Recommended dosage: 1,000 mg daily.*

- **Tripterygium wilfordii (TG):** Also known as thundergod vine, this is a well-known Chinese herbal medicine with the active ingredient celastrol. It has been evaluated in many clinical trials and found to be effective in treating psoriasis, lupus, rheumatoid arthritis, and ulcerative colitis, among others.[39] In RA, it prevents bone and cartilage erosion, and in Crohn's disease, it was found to be as effective as the common drug azathioprine in preventing recurrence after surgery. It works by blocking multiple inflammation pathways and steers T cell polarization away from Th17 production.[40] *Recommended dosage: Since TG is not standardized, there are no absolute recommended doses, although the effective dose in Crohn's patients was 1.5 mg/kg of body weight. I would consult with a Chinese medicine herbalist to get your proper dosage.*

- **Ursolic acid:** This is another compound that is gaining interest because of its effectiveness in shutting down auto-immune disease. In animal studies, it was found to reduce autoimmune arthritis by decreasing markers of disease and Th17 cells.[41] Ursolic acid is a natural component found in apple peels but also in herbs such as oregano, basil, thyme, and rosemary. *Recommended dosage: 300 mg daily.*

Because each of us has a unique immune system imbalance, your Immune Restoration Plan should be tailored to your needs, which is why the next chapter might just be the most important one in this book. So many health books throw pages and pages of advice at you—pages filled with supplements and foods and life-style practice and exercises—but then give you no way to zero in on what you're actually going to do. I don't expect you to follow every suggestion and take every supplement in the Toolkits. In fact, you'll get the best results if you choose one suggestion from each of the sleep, stress, gut health, toxins, and nutrition chapters and incorporate these five interventions into your daily routine. In addition, start three of the supplements that correspond to your Immunotype. I'm going to ask you to do this for at least thirty days before you judge your results. Once you get comfortable in your new routine, you can add more Toolkit suggestions and sup-plements to your routine.

CHAPTER 11

The Immune Restoration Plan at a Glance

My goal is for you to take all the data from Part II of this book and put it into action so you can feel vibrant, confident, and secure about your future health. But admittedly, that was a *lot* of info, which is why I created this chapter. Here, I'll ask you to fill out an Immune Restoration Plan at a Glance. It will help you pick action items from each chapter—on sleep, stress, gut health, toxins, and nutrition—as well as supplements to incorporate into your first thirty days on the Immune Restoration Plan. That way, you're clear about your path forward and can refer to the At a Glance anytime in those thirty days if you need to refresh your memory or motivate yourself to stick to your action items.

You'll notice that some of the boxes are blank—no, that's not a mistake! I've filled in the initial action item that everyone with that Immunotype should take for the first thirty days; then I've left blank space for you to fill in the one recommendation from each of the chapters in Part II that feels most doable for you.

Remember, if you have more than one Immunotype, follow the plan for your primary Immunotype first. You can always retake the Four Immunotypes Quiz at the end to see if your primary Immunotype has changed and then tackle that plan next!

Why have I done this? Because personalization goes far beyond Immunotypes. We all have different habits, challenges, schedules, budgets, and priorities. I'm not here to give you a prescriptive plan that you have to uproot your entire life to follow—I'm here to help you rebalance your immune system in the way that works best for you and doesn't make you feel like you're swimming upstream!

CREATING YOUR PERSONALIZED IMMUNE RESTORATION PLAN

To create your Immune Restoration Plan at a Glance, first find the chart that corresponds to your primary Immunotype. Look at the information I've already filled out for you. Then go back and read the Toolkits from Part II, select the one recommendation from each Toolkit that feels the most doable (for thirty days), and write it in the blank space. You may be tempted to adopt more than one Toolkit action item for each lifestyle pillar, but I urge you to concentrate on one of each for the first thirty days so you can make them into habits. Then, if you feel comfortable, add a second action item for each fundamental pillar for the next thirty days, and so on. Remember, you can start up to three supplements in the first thirty days and continue for at least sixty days before adding more supplements into the mix.

Weak Immunotype — At a Glance

Goal: To boost the immune system by increasing Th1 cells and cytokines as well as bolstering B cell activity and production of antibodies and natural killer cells.

Fundamental Pillar: Sleep	Supplements (first 60 days)
- Avoid all blue light for 2 hours before bed	1) Melatonin, 3 mg one hour before bedtime
-	2)
-	3)
Lifestyle Pillars:	

How I'm decreasing my stress (pick 1 Toolkit item):

How I'm investing in my gut health (pick 1 Toolkit item):

How I'm detoxifying my life (pick 1 Toolkit item):

How I'm improving my nutrition (pick 1 Toolkit item):

Smoldering Immunotype — At a Glance

Goal: To dismantle the causes of inflammation and accelerate its resolution to avoid a cycle of chronic immune activation.

Fundamental Pillar: Nutrition	Supplements (first 60 days)
- Reduce your intake of added sugars	1) Curcumin, 1,000 mg twice a day with food
	2)
	3)
Lifestyle Pillars:	

How I'm optimizing my sleep (pick 1 Toolkit item):

How I'm decreasing stress (pick 1 Toolkit item):

How I'm investing in my gut health (pick 1 Toolkit item):

How I'm detoxifying my life (pick 1 Toolkit item):

Hyperactive Immunotype—At a Glance

Goal: To boost the immune system by increasing Th1 cells and cytokines as well as bolstering B cell activity and production of antibodies and natural killer cells.

Fundamental Pillar: Toxins	Supplements (first 60 days):
- Clean up your cleaning products	1) Quercetin, 1,000 mg twice a day with food
-	2)
-	3)
Lifestyle Pillars:	

How I'm optimizing my sleep (pick 1 Toolkit item):

How I'm decreasing stress (pick 1 Toolkit item):

How I'm investing in my gut health (pick 1 Toolkit item):

How I'm improving my nutrition (pick 1 Toolkit item):

Misguided Immunotype—At a Glance

Goal: To dampen excessive inflammation; block damaging Th17 cell activity, which perpetuates tissue destruction in autoimmune disease; and hit the off switch of an overexuberant immune response, by increasing regulatory T cells.

Fundamental Pillar: Gut health	Supplements (first 60 days):
- Do an elimination diet	1) Vitamin D, at least 2,000 IU a day, with food
-	2)
-	3)
Lifestyle Pillars:	

How I'm investing in sleep (pick 1 Toolkit item):

How I'm decreasing stress (pick 1 Toolkit item):

How I'm detoxifying my life (pick 1 Toolkit item):

How I'm improving my nutrition (pick 1 Toolkit item):

WHAT TO EXPECT AS YOU START YOUR IMMUNE RESTORATION PLAN

Once you've filled out your Immune Restoration Plan at a Glance, you're ready to dive into your first thirty days. Is there anything else you should know before you get started?

First, I recommend that you use a journal or digital calendar to track your progress and make note of how you feel as you progress. If you're not paying close attention, it can be easy to overlook small incremental improvements in your health and well-being. Keeping a log of your symptoms can help you notice these small improvements and stop you from getting discouraged.

Second, keep in mind that it's taken months if not years for your Immunotype to develop, so it's important to be patient. This Immune Restoration Plan lasts thirty days, but it's not a detox or a cleanse; it's designed as a jumping-off point for long-term lifestyle change. I recommend focusing less on your goals in the first thirty days and more on establishing habits that feel doable. Continue to do that and over time you'll notice your body becoming less inflamed, your energy increasing, and your symptoms improving.

I know this may seem slow at first, but if you do it this way, new habits are more likely to stick. After all, radical transformation doesn't happen overnight; small changes add up, and before you know it you'll be feeling amazing. In fact, studies show that it takes an average of sixty-six days to form a new habit and make it stick! Most of us have some deeply ingrained not-so-healthy habits that we've been practicing for a long time, so be kind to yourself. It's really the compounding interest of your daily habits over time that shapes your future. As James Clear, the author of *Atomic Habits*, states, "Habits often appear to make no difference until you cross a critical threshold and unlock a new level of performance." I see the same thing every day with my clients. Positive results can seem far out of reach when you feel terrible and have felt terrible for so long. Many of my patients are confused about what to do, and they haven't been given hope by their doctors. Perhaps, like you, they tried some diet they read about on a blog or took some immune-"boosting" vitamins for a while, but they gave up because they didn't notice any difference. I get it! That's why I've distilled what I know to be the most impactful steps you can take to revive and balance your immune system.

I wish I could say there was an overnight hack or magic pill to instantaneously transform your immune system's health. There isn't. But if you follow these steps and are patient with yourself and your body, changes will happen. I've seen this time and time again in my patients who have broken through their thresholds by being persistent and trusting in their bodies' innate capacity to heal.

LAB WORK AND THE FOUR IMMUNOTYPES

You've taken the Four Immunotypes Quiz, and now you're pretty clear on your primary and maybe even secondary Immunotype. You might be wondering, is there a way to confirm that your quiz results are accurate? In my office, I typically diagnose an Immunotype through the patient's health history and current symptoms—similar to taking the Four Immunotypes Quiz—but I also confirm it with bloodwork. And while I obviously can't order lab work for every single person who reads this book, I can give you the tests I would run for each Immunotype so that you're armed with the right information and can work with your health care professional to confirm your Immunotype. This isn't a requirement, but it can be helpful if you score high on more than one Immunotype, have a tie between two, or just want to confirm your results. Getting lab tests that confirm your Immunotype can also help you stay motivated to keep up with healthy lifestyle changes and can act as a way to track your progress.

So, without further ado, here are the lab tests I would recommend for each Immunotype.

Lab Work for the Weak Immunotype:

1. A complete blood count: This is referred to as a CBC and is routinely run as a screening test for anemia. It also measures your total white blood cell count, which includes your neutrophils, monocytes (baby macrophages), and lymphocytes (collectively, your T and B cells). If you have a low white blood cell count overall or low percentages of lymphocytes and neutrophils, this can tip you off that something is amiss. I recommend that *all* Immunotypes have a complete blood count.

2. The CD4/CD8 ratio: This test measures the ratio of your helper T cells to killer T cells. During the AIDS crisis, low helper T cell counts indicated that the virus was destroying the immune system, and it was an ominous sign. We also know that a lagging CD4 number is a sign that the immune system is aging faster than it should. The corollary is that a normal CD4 count in the elderly is a sign of a robust immune system. In fact, a study in Sweden of healthy hundred-year-olds found that they had CD4/CD8 ratios like young people![1] *Normal range: 1.5 to 2.5 or more.*

3. Total immunoglobulins: This is a measurement of your total antibody supply. It doesn't tell you if you're protected

against specific infections, just how much rough material you have to work with. Although it's rare, adults can be relatively healthy throughout life but then be found to have low or borderline levels of total IgG or IgA. This is important, as IgG is the class of antibodies that protects us long-term from infections, and IgA is the antibody that protects the surface of our respiratory tract and GI tract. Low IgG can be very serious, but it can be treated long-term with intravenous immunoglobulin from donors if necessary. Low IgA is not treatable, but it's not as serious, and knowing your status allows you to take extra precautions against getting sick.

4. Epstein-Barr virus (EBV) antibodies: About 90 percent of the world has at one time been infected with EBV, the virus responsible for mononucleosis, usually as a child or teenager. Therefore, most of us will have antibodies to EBV, even if we don't remember getting sick. This is totally normal. However, an elevated result in a test called early antigen D can mean the virus is reactivated and replicating, indicating a weakness in our immune system's ability to keep it at bay.

Lab Work for a Smoldering Immunotype

1. C-reactive protein (CRP): This is one of the best tests we have for inflammation. Specifically request the high-sensitivity CRP. It's a more sensitive test, especially for inflammation in blood vessels. It tests for levels of the proinflammatory cytokine IL-6. *Normal range: less than 3.0 mg/L.*

2. Hemoglobin A1c and fasting insulin: A single test of your glucose level may be normal on the day that you get it tested. Hemoglobin A1c is a far better test because it gives

you an average of the past ninety days of your blood sugar. Fasting insulin goes one step further. Elevations in fasting insulin even with a normal blood sugar may indicate that your pancreas is working overtime, pumping out insulin in an effort to keep your blood sugar down. Both of these blood tests are easy to get. *Normal range: hemoglobin A1c, less than 5.7 percent; fasting insulin, 3 to 8 uIU/mL.*

3. Oxidized LDL: High levels in this test indicate that cholesterol particles are damaged or oxidized. Oxidized LDL stimulates inflammation especially in blood vessels, and it's a good predictive test for heart attacks and coronary artery disease in general. *Normal range: less than 60 U/L.*

Lab Work for a Hyperactive Immunotype

The lab tests for a Hyperactive Immunotype are mostly looking for signs of Th2 dominance, which can be revealed by the following tests:

1. Eosinophil count: This is measured in a routine CBC, and when elevated can be a sign of allergies or a parasite infection. *Anything above 3 percent is abnormal.*

2. IgE immunoglobulin: When this is elevated, it's always correlated with the Hyperactive Immunotype. *Normal range: less than 114 kU/L.*

3. Parasites: Because of the way parasites replicate, they're often missed in a stool test, even if you are infected. However, a stool test showing parasites indicates a shift to Th2 dominance.

What Can You Really Learn from a Stool Test?

The information you get from stool tests varies greatly among labs. Most national laboratory chains do stool testing for different bacterial infections, like *H. pylori*, salmonella, *C. difficile*, parasites, and some viruses. However, some specialty lab companies have much more comprehensive, all-in-one tests to evaluate what's really going on. Some benefits to getting one of these tests are that you will learn:

- how inflamed your gut is.
- how well you digest fat, protein, and carbs.
- how many good bacteria you have, and what their patterns are.
- how many pathogenic bacteria and parasites you have.

Overall, these lab tests do an in-depth analysis of your total gut health, which is really important information to have when you're trying to transform your immune health.

Lab Work for a Misguided Immunotype

1. Complete blood count: As I discussed in the Weak Immunotype lab test section, this simple blood test can give you so much information. A change you might see that hints at increased Th17 activity is a high neutrophil count. These white blood cells are always involved in tissue destruction.

2. Vitamin D level (25-hydroxy vitamin D): Because vitamin D is such an important immune modulator, and vitamin D deficiency has been associated with autoimmune

disease, you want to have robust levels, between 50 and 80 ng/ml, for optimal health. You'll often be told that your levels are normal just because they fall inside the wider lab range of 30 to 100 nm/ml. Levels closer to 30 are deemed "adequate" for bone health, but to optimize immune health you want to aim higher. Studies on prevention of viral infection have indicated that higher levels of vitamin D are necessary.[2] In fact, low vitamin D levels have been correlated with higher mortality from influenza and COVID-19.[3] There is a risk of hypervitaminosis D if you take too much, but this is rare. I recommend having your vitamin D levels checked eight weeks after supplementation to make sure you're in range.

3. C-reactive protein (CRP): As with the Smoldering Immunotype, I always want to measure the level of CRP because it goes up with increasing activity of Th17 cells and the destructive cytokine IL-6. It gives us some sense of the level of inflammation.

4. Common autoimmune antibodies: I run a panel testing several of these antibodies, which may show up years before someone is symptomatic.

    a. ANA: One of the most important is ANA (antinuclear antibody), which is an antibody to the contents of the nucleus of our cells. ANA is often elevated in lupus and several other diseases.

    b. Anti-TPO and anti-thyroglobulin: Anti-TPO and anti-thyroglobulin antibodies are elevated in autoimmune thyroid disease.

    c. Celiac antibodies: Celiac disease screening is important, including for tissue transglutaminase antibodies (tTG-IgA) and IgA endomysial antibody (EMA), as well as levels of immunoglobulins A and G. If total

IgA and total IgG are low, not only does this indicate an underlying immune deficiency, but it also makes the screening tests for celiac and infections less reliable.

d. Virus antibodies: Antibody levels to viruses in the herpes family, like Epstein-Barr virus (EBV), herpes simplex virus (HSV), and cytomegalovirus (CMV), may be elevated in the Misguided Immunotype, and will continue to propel an inflammatory response.

5. IgG food sensitivity test and a microbiome stool test: These may be harder to get through your primary doctor, but you can get them through a functional medicine practitioner. Patients with autoimmune disease have leaky gut issues and frequent food sensitivities. It's crucial to identify and stop eating the foods you're sensitive to, as they only fuel inflammation. Lastly, a comprehensive stool test can detect inflammation and hidden infections in the gut like parasites and *H. pylori,* as well as the pattern of healthy microflora. These factors play a huge role in triggering disease and maintaining symptoms.

These tests can be extremely helpful, but I want to be clear that *you do not need them as proof before you start taking major steps to squelch your immune imbalances.* Keep in mind that while most of the tests will be available through mainstream labs, others may only be run through specialty labs and may not be covered by insurance.

IMMUNE RESTORATION PLAN
TROUBLESHOOTING

As you begin your Immune Restoration Plan, you're bound to run into challenges, whether with the plan itself or with staying motivated. Having helped many patients through very similar lifestyle changes, I've tried to predict some of the issues you may run into below and have outlined my best advice for how to move past them!

What to do if you can't stay motivated

If you're having trouble completing the Immune Restoration Plan, I'd recommend a few different things. But first, I understand that change can be hard, especially around things that may give us short-term comfort, like the foods we eat. Habits are deeply ingrained, so it can feel overwhelming and even anxiety-provoking to make changes. If you're having trouble completing the first thirty days, I suggest:

- Phone a friend: Doing the Immune Restoration Plan with a friend can help you stay motivated and make it a whole lot more fun. Plus, you'll be helping one of your loved ones improve their health!
- Lean on a health coach: Health coaches are some of the most underrated health professionals out there, and they can help you stay motivated and on task. Just make sure they have some type of official certification and training ("health coach" is not a regulated term, and anyone can call themselves one, even if they don't have any official training). The best thing about health coaches is that many of them can do phone or virtual sessions, so you can find one who feels like a good fit without being restricted by location.
- Write down your "why": There's a reason why you picked up this book. Maybe you're sick of getting every cough and cold that goes around the office; maybe you're suffering daily from pain from an autoimmune condition; maybe

your allergies are getting so bad you're considering moving to a different state. Whatever your why, write it down in a letter to yourself and read it once a week. It will reconnect you to your motivations and help you keep the faith!

What to do if you're not sure your Immunotype is correct

I'd recommend retaking the Four Immunotypes Quiz, trying to answer as honestly as you can. You can get the recommended lab work done, which will give you extra information. You can also do all of the recommended interventions from Chapters 5 through 9—they'll really help every Immunotype. Start the specific supplements recommended for your Immunotype; however, if after sixty days you don't feel any improvement in your health, talk with a health professional about a further evaluation.

What to do if you feel worse after starting your Immune Restoration Plan

It's possible to feel worse before you get better, but this should stay within reason. Sometimes when you cut out foods like sugar, wheat, dairy, and caffeinated beverages, you can actually go through a bit of a withdrawal. You may feel a little achy, irritable, and tired, and you may crave sugar or these other foods for a few days to a week. That's normal! What's not normal is pain, increased GI issues, or an exacerbation of symptoms, especially symptoms of a chronic disease. If any of that happens, stop all supplements and consult with your doctor.

What to do if you're not sure about supplements

Supplements have developed a bit of a reputation in recent years, and admittedly, there are people in the supplement industry who are much more interested in making money off you than they are in supporting your health. That said, there are brands that are committed to creating the highest-quality products, and I do believe that supplements are an important part of rebalancing an Immunotype. If you decide to forgo supplements, try to eat as many food sources of that nutrient and as many fruits and vegetables as possible. You'll still get tremendous benefits.

What to do if you don't have the support of your doctor

Unfortunately, many doctors will tell you that nutrition and lifestyle changes will not influence your health. If your doctor tries to discourage you from making healthy lifestyle changes, go back to the section in Chapter 1 titled "The Good News—Nurture > Nature," where I list statistics about how a healthy lifestyle can, unarguably, prevent or reduce health issues. A good doctor will support your efforts to live a healthier lifestyle, and if they don't, it might be time to look for a second opinion!

YOU'VE DONE YOUR FIRST THIRTY DAYS, NOW WHAT?

How do you feel? Pat yourself on the back for completing thirty days of tackling bad habits and picking up new ones. Take this time to assess how you feel in general. Have you noticed any changes in your energy, mood, digestion, or other symptoms? Do you feel less inflamed? Go back to your Toolkits and grab a new lifestyle change from each category to work on this month; just don't let the others slide. If you had any abnormal lab test results before you started the program, get them checked again after sixty days, especially if you're taking supplements such as vitamin

D. If you're still having significant symptoms of inflammation, allergy, autoimmune disease, or illness, you can return to the supplement list to make sure you're taking the maximum dosage. In addition, you can add one or two more supplements for your type.

After the first thirty days, I recommend retaking the Four Immunotypes Quiz to see how much you've improved. But my hope is that you don't need a quiz to tell you you're feeling better. My hope is that you notice those improvements in your energy, mood, pain, other symptoms, and overall health. The Immune Restoration Plan was designed to be sustainable, so technically, you never have to stop doing the plan! It can be done again and again, with you retaking the quiz regularly to see if your primary Immunotype has changed.

The Secret to Lifelong Immune Balance

I've thought long and hard about the last words I want to say in this book, which is the culmination of years of research and learning and experience. And this is it: Your immune system is constantly changing and adapting, and you have the opportunity to make tremendous changes to improve your physical state every day when you choose what to eat, how much to sleep and exercise, and how to manage stress. Whether you feel inflamed, have allergies or autoimmune disease, or are always tired and sick, following the Immune Restoration Plan is going to get you on the road to healing.

This is what I teach my patients every day, and now that you've read this book, you have the tools and knowledge to keep your immune system running like a well-oiled, efficient fighting machine. Maybe you've started to make changes in your life by incorporating a few of the steps from each of the Immune Restoration Toolkits; perhaps you're sporting your blue-light-blocking glasses every night, taking curcumin daily, dedicating yourself to fifteen minutes of meditation a day, and, dare I say it, regularly eating greens with your breakfast. Whatever steps you're taking, keep going. Over time, your body will pay you back in spades with better immune health, more energy, and less inflammation, aches, and pains.

One of my main goals in writing this book was to demystify the immune system, because it can be so intimidating to the average person. I mean, even the experts don't have all the answers! I am still awestruck by the intelligence of this system that finds its home in all of our bodies. Every day, we discover more and more secrets to immunity that inch us closer and closer to maximizing health and living well longer. Just some of the discoveries made in the past few years are a new type of brain-protective macrophage that may help prevent Alzheimer's disease, new ways to use nano-technology to increase immune tolerance and reduce food allergies, and of course the rise of mRNA vaccines to bring down a worldwide pandemic in record time. We're also making tremendous strides in understanding how our emotional state, childhood upbringing, and social connections impact how resilient we are, and how these factors inform our immune systems. At a time when there is much social upheaval and turmoil in the world, understanding this relationship is crucial to our health.

Scientists and citizens alike need to continue the quest to understand how climate change, population growth, destruction of animal habitats, and environmental toxins are all connected to our immune health. We know that "novel" viruses are new to us but have been lurking on the earth in other hosts for hundreds of years, slowly replicating and mutating until an environmental shift occurs and spillover happens, placing us right in the viruses' path. We also know, as I have touched on, that massive environmental pollution is changing how our immune systems develop and how they function throughout life. We even inherit epigenetic changes from our ancestors caused by environmental factors that have occurred generations before. Our bodies adapt as best they can to changes in our ecosystem and to outside threats, but they can only do that so quickly. Evolutionary adaptation takes millennia, and our planet is rapidly changing to the point that we're struggling to keep up. I say this not to depress you, but instead to impress upon you that our immune systems are constantly influenced by the changes that are going on inside and outside our bodies. The immune system has an incredible capacity to learn and will continue to do so as we meet new challenges—but we need to help it along by giving it support and protection in how we live our lives.

I want to give you hope and empower you to take charge of your health, however frustrating it may feel at this moment. Because the immune system is so complex, it may seem as if you don't have control over what happens to you. In fact, one of the things that bothers me the most is when a patient has been told by another practitioner that there's nothing they can do for them other than to prescribe medication and urge them to accept their new fate. This is simply wrong; it's not only a disservice to the patient, but to my mind also shows a lack of desire or duty for that practitioner to learn. We must think outside the box and not just cling to approaches that worked twenty years ago. With reasoning like that we wouldn't have iPads, Uber, Venmo, Alexa, or many other technological advances that have changed our lives.

I believe in modern medicine immensely, but not at the expense of the integral healing power of the human body. In her book *Radical Remission,* Dr. Kelly A. Turner interviewed hundreds of practitioners and their patients who had survived cancer against all odds after conventional treatments had failed them.

She found that these survivors tended to have these traits and habits:

1. They changed their diet.
2. They took control of their health.
3. They followed their intuition.
4. They used herbs and supplements.
5. They released suppressed emotions.
6. They increased positive emotions.
7. They embraced social support.
8. They deepened their spiritual connection.
9. They had strong reasons for living.

My hope is that with a deeper understanding of your own immune system and where its weaknesses and strengths lie, with the knowledge of your Immunotype, and with a tailored plan for nourishing, protecting, calming, strengthening, and redirecting your immune system, you too can attain immune balance to live a long, healthy life.

Acknowledgments

The seeds were planted for me to write this book before any of us knew of the global pandemic that was about to erupt. But in a way, the fact that a tiny virus could bring the world to a screeching halt inspired me even more to keep writing about a subject that is so important and essential to all of us—our personal immune systems.

Numerous individuals have played a part in helping me accomplish my dream of writing a book. I want to specifically thank a few of them, without whom this never would have happened.

Firstly, I wouldn't have been granted this opportunity without my superlative agent, Heather Jackson. I feel so blessed that the universe conspired for us to cross paths and for you to ask the question "Have you ever thought about writing a book?" Your steadfast encouragement, as well as your uncanny ability to help me visualize my ideas, has been invaluable. Thank you for being my navigator and always looking out for my best interests.

To my amazing editor, Tracy Behar at Little, Brown Spark: I feel like I won the lottery. You were willing to take a chance on my manuscript, and me, and I feel so fortunate to have had the opportunity to create this book with your guidance. Your razor-sharp editing and feedback have been priceless.

To the talented Gretchen Lidicker, collaborator extraordinaire: Thank you for keeping me on track and making me laugh when I was feeling overwhelmed. I am indebted to you and your experience in helping me organize, refine, and shape an often-complicated subject into a wonderful book.

To the gifted designer Marlene Large, who created the excellent illustrations in this book: Thank you for making the Four Immunotypes come to life on the page.

To Dr. Firdaus Dharbar, for being so kind and generous in sharing your research and knowledge with me: It's scientists like you who are so crucial in advancing the science of immunology every day.

To my exceptional team of superwomen at the Moday Center, who kept us afloat and thriving through this tumultuous year: Thanks to Kayleigh McClory for being an incredible nutritionist and creating social media content that is out of this world. Thanks to Kristie Depippo for being the glue that keeps us all together and running like a well-oiled machine. Thank you both for your flexibility during this crazy time. I couldn't have done it without you.

To the inspirational Dr. Katie Takayasu: I am so blessed that we found each other in Arizona as integrative medicine fellows. Thank you for your sage advice, the sanity check-ins, and true friendship.

Thanks to Jason and Colleen Wachob and the mindbodygreen team for spreading the wellness message to the world and for championing me and other functional medicine practitioners along the way.

I am indebted to the numerous doctors, scientists, and other practitioners whom I have learned from over the years. I am standing on many shoulders. Whether in real life or online, I am constantly motivated and supported by so many brilliant trailblazers. A special thanks to Dr. Grace Liu, aka the Gut Goddess, who taught me so much about the gut microbiome—you are a rock star.

To my patients, who are also my teachers, you are why I do what I do. You inspire me every day. Thank you.

I am so very grateful for the many friends who have emailed, texted, and checked in on me during the writing of this book. In particular, Sam Wegman: Our frequent pep talks and your unwavering reassurance over the past year have helped me more than you know.

To my incredible AFL sisters and SS tribe: We may never have met in real life, but your nurturing words, wisdom, and laughter have changed me for the better. My heartfelt thanks to each and every one of you.

I am fortunate to have amazing siblings and extended family who are always championing me—especially my parents, Peggy and Donald Moday, who always encouraged me to write and to forge my own path. You will always be my biggest cheerleaders.

And lastly, to my incredible partner, Erica, whose patience, love, and understanding are immeasurable. You were there to lift my confidence when it was waning, make me dinner, give me space, and remind me to have fun. You made this crazy year actually pretty amazing. Thank you for being my rock.

Resources

People often ask me, "How do I find a functional medicine doctor or specialist to work with?" There are several excellent training programs in functional and integrative medicine, and practitioners have varied backgrounds, expertise, and levels of training.

Here are some good places to start:

The Institute for Functional Medicine. Look in their practitioner database for a "certified" practitioner. https://www.ifm.org/find-a-practitioner/

The American Academy of Anti-Aging Medicine (A4M) is the established global leader for continuing medical education in longevity medicine, metabolic resilience, and whole-person care. https://www.a4m.com/find-a-doctor.html

LAB COMPANIES

There are many excellent companies that run a myriad of functional health labs useful in assessing the systems discussed in this book. These are the ones I use regularly and recommend. Most if not all of these lab companies require that the tests be ordered and interpreted by a registered practitioner.

Microbiome/GI health:

- Trio-Smart tests https://www.triosmartbreath.com
- Commonwealth Diagnostics International: https://commdx .com
- Doctor's Data: www.Doctorsdata.com
- Genova Diagnostics: https://www.gdx.net
- Diagnostic Solutions Laboratory: https://www.diagnostic solutionslab.com

Micronutrient testing:

- Spectracell Laboratories: https://www.spectracell.com
- Vibrant America: https://www.vibrant-america.com/micro nutrient

Stress hormone testing:

- Precision Analytical DUTCH test (dried urine test for total comprehensive hormones): https://dutchtest.com

Food sensitivity and autoimmune testing:

- VibrantWellness: https://www.vibrant-wellness.com/tests /food-sensitivity
- Cyrex Laboratories: https://www.cyrexlabs.com

Testing for organic toxins, heavy metals, and mold:

- Great Plains Laboratory: https://www.greatplainslaboratory .com
- Quicksilver Scientific: https://www.quicksilverscientific.com /testing-products

RECOMMENDED PRODUCTS

Sleep:

Blue-light-blocking glasses:

- Swanwick: https://www.swanwicksleep.com
- Bedtime Bulb: https://bedtimebulb.com

Blue-light-blocking applications and websites:

- F.lux: https://justgetflux.com
- Twilight: https://twilight.urbandroid.org

Sleep trackers:

- Oura Ring: https://ouraring.com

Stress management:

Meditation apps:

- Calm: https://www.calm.com
- InsightTimer: https://insighttimer.com
- Headspace: https://www.headspace.com
- Breethe: heeps://breethe.com

Breath techniques:

- Four-seven-eight breath: https://www.drweil.com/videos
  -features/videos/breathing-exercises-4-7-8-breath

Emotional Freedom Technique/tapping:

- Gary Craig Official EFT Training Centers: https://www
  .emofree.com
- The Tapping Solution: https://www.thetappingsolution.com

Environmental health:

To find nontoxic personal care and cleaning products, a safe sunscreen guide, and tap-water quality maps, go to the Environmental Working Group website: https://www.ewg.org.

Air purifiers:

- Austin Air Systems: https://austinair.com
- Coway Air Purifier: https://www.cowayairpurifiers.com
- IQAir: https://www.iqair.com

Clean water systems:

- Aquasana: https://www.aquasana.com
- Berkey Filters: https://www.berkeyfilters.com

Supplements:

There are many excellent supplement companies out there.
- Pure Encapsulations: https://www.pureencapsulations.com
- Thorne: https://www.thorne.com
- Metagenics: https://www.metagenics.com
- Designs for Health: https://www.designsforhealth.com
- Xymogen: https://www.xymogen.com
- Mushroom Revival: https://www.mushroomrevival.com

For independent reviews of many other supplement companies, go to ConsumerLab: https://www.consumerlab.com.

Notes

Chapter 1: The Immune Dysfunction Crisis

1. Marineli F, Tsoucalas G, Karamanou M, Androutsos G. Mary Mallon (1869–1938) and the history of typhoid fever. *Ann Gastroenterol.* 2013; 26(2):132–134.

2. Arias E. United States life tables, 2008. Natl Vital Stat Rep. 2012 Sep 24; 61(3):1–63. PMID: 24974590.

3. CDC. Heart Disease Facts. Centers for Disease Control and Prevention. Published September 8, 2020. Accessed April 25, 2021. https://www.cdc .gov/heartdisease/facts.htm.

4. Centers for Disease Control and Prevention. National Diabetes Statistics Report, 2020. Atlanta: Centers for Disease Control and Prevention, U.S. Dept of Health and Human Services, 2020.

5. https://www.cdc.gov/media/releases/2017/p0718-diabetes-report.html.

6. https://www.alz.org/alzheimers-dementia/facts-figures.

7. https://www.cdc.gov/nchs/data/hestat/obesity_adult_07_08/obesity _adult_07_08.pdf.

8. The State of Mental Health in America. Mental Health America. Accessed April 25, 2021. https://www.mhanational.org/issues/state-mental-health -america#Key.

9. Autoimmune Diseases. National Institute of Environmental Health Sciences. Accessed April 25, 2021. https://www.niehs.nih.gov/health/topics /conditions/autoimmune/index.cfm.

10. Anderson G. Chronic care: making the case for ongoing care. Princeton (NJ): Robert Wood Johnson Foundation; 2010. http://www.rwjf.org

/content/dam/farm/reports/reports/2010/rwjf54583. Accessed September 1, 2014.

11. Martin CB, Hales CM, Gu Q, Ogden CL. Prescription drug use in the United States, 2015–2016. NCHS Data Brief, no 334. Hyattsville, MD: National Center for Health Statistics. 2019.

12. https://www.cdc.gov/nchs/fastats/drug-use-therapeutic.htm.

13. Brody DJ, Gu Q. Antidepressant use among adults: United States, 2015–2018. NCHS Data Brief, no 377. Hyattsville, MD: National Center for Health Statistics. 2020.

14. Wongrakpanich S, Wongrakpanich A, Melhado K, Rangaswami J. A Comprehensive Review of Non-Steroidal Anti-Inflammatory Drug Use in the Elderly. *Aging Dis.* 2018; 9(1):143–150. Published 2018 Feb 1. doi:10.14336/AD.2017.0306.

15. Centers for Disease Control and Prevention. 2018 Annual Surveillance Report of Drug-Related Risks and Outcomes—United States. Surveillance Special Report. Centers for Disease Control and Prevention, U.S. Department of Health and Human Services. Published August 31, 2018.

16. Salami JA, Warraich H, Valero-Elizondo J, et al. National Trends in Statin Use and Expenditures in the US Adult Population from 2002 to 2013: Insights from the Medical Expenditure Panel Survey. *JAMA Cardiol.* 2017; 2(1):56–65. doi:10.1001/jamacardio.2016.4700.

17. https://medicine.wustl.edu/news/popular-heartburn-drugs-linked-to-fatal-heart-disease-chronic-kidney-disease-stomach-cancer/#:~:text=More%20than%2015%20million%20Americans%20have%20prescriptions%20for%20PPIs.

18. https://www.drugwatch.com/featured/is-your-heartburn-drug-necessary/#:~:text=PPIs%20come%20with%20rare%20but,even%20when%20they%20shouldn't.

19. Villarroel MA, Blackwell DL, Jen A. Tables of Summary Health Statistics for U.S. Adults: 2018 National Health Interview Survey. National Center for Health Statistics. 2019. Available from: http://www.cdc.gov/nchs/nhis/SHS/tables.htm. SOURCE: NCHS, National Health Interview Survey, 2018.

20. Felger JC. Role of Inflammation in Depression and Treatment Implications. *Handb Exp Pharmacol.* 2019; 250:255–286. doi:10.1007/164_2018_166.

21. Strachan DP. Hay fever, hygiene, and household size. *BMJ.* 1989; 299(6710): 1259–1260. doi:10.1136/bmj.299.6710.1259.

22. Bloomfield SF, Rook GA, Scott EA, Shanahan F, Stanwell-Smith R, Turner P. Time to abandon the hygiene hypothesis: new perspectives on allergic disease, the human microbiome, infectious disease prevention and the role of targeted hygiene. *Perspect Public Health*. 2016; 136(4):213–224.

23. https://www.hsph.harvard.edu/news/hsph-in-the-news/doctors-nutrition -education/#:~:text=%E2%80%9CToday%2C%20most%20medical%20 schools%20in,in%20nutrition%2C%20it's%20a%20scandal.

24. http://www.imperial.ac.uk/news/177778/eating-more-fruits-vegetables -prevent-millions/.

25. Liu YZ, Wang YX, Jiang CL. Inflammation: The Common Pathway of Stress-Related Diseases. *Front Hum Neurosci*. 2017; 11:316. Published 2017 Jun 20. doi:10.3389/fnhum.2017.00316.

26. https://health.clevelandclinic.org/how-environmental-toxins-can-impact -your-health/.

27. Yang Q, Zhang Z, Gregg EW, Flanders WD, Merritt R, Hu FB. Added sugar intake and cardiovascular diseases mortality among US adults. JAMA Intern Med. 2014;174(4):516–524. doi:10.1001/jamainternmed.2013 .13563.

28. Moling O, Gandini L. Sugar and the Mosaic of Autoimmunity. *Am J Case Rep*. 2019; 20:1364–1368. Published 2019 Sep 15. doi:10.12659/AJCR .915703.

29. Prossegger J, Huber D, Grafetstätter C, et al. Winter Exercise Reduces Allergic Airway Inflammation: A Randomized Controlled Study. *Int J Environ Res Public Health*. 2019; 16(11):2040. Published 2019 Jun 8. doi:10.3390/ijerph16112040.

Chapter 2: Immunity 101 — Understanding Your Immune Army

1. Carvalheiro H, Duarte C, Silva-Cardoso S, da Silva JAP, Souto-Carneiro, MM. (2015), CD8+ T Cell Profiles in Patients with Rheumatoid Arthritis and Their Relationship to Disease Activity. *Arthritis & Rheumatology, 67:* 363–371.

2. Pender MP. "CD8+ T-Cell Deficiency, Epstein-Barr Virus Infection, Vitamin D Deficiency, and Steps to Autoimmunity: A Unifying Hypothesis." *Autoimmune Diseases*, vol. 2012, Article ID 189096, 16 pages, 2012.

Chapter 3: Chronic Inflammation—The Heart of Immune System Imbalance

1. Ciaccia L. Fundamentals of Inflammation. *Yale J Biol Med.* 2011; 84(1): 64–65.

2. Micha R, Mozaffarian D. Saturated fat and cardiometabolic risk factors, coronary heart disease, stroke, and diabetes: a fresh look at the evidence. *Lipids.* 2010; 45(10):893–905. doi:10.1007/s11745-010-3393-4.

3. Dhaka V, Gulia N, Ahlawat KS, Khatkar BS. Trans fats-sources, health risks and alternative approach: A review. *Journal of Food Science and Technology.* 2011 Oct;48(5):534–541. doi: 10.1007/s13197-010-0225-8.

4. Yang Q, Zhang Z, Gregg EW, Flanders WD, Merritt R, Hu FB. Added Sugar Intake and Cardiovascular Diseases Mortality Among US Adults. *JAMA Intern Med.* 2014; 174(4):516–524. doi:10.1001/jamainternmed.2013 .13563.

5. Singer K, DelProposto J, Morris DL, et al. Diet-induced obesity promotes myelopoiesis in hematopoietic stem cells. *Mol Metab.* 2014; 3(6):664–675. Published 2014 Jul 10. doi:10.1016/j.molmet.2014.06.005.

6. Basaranoglu M, Basaranoglu G, Bugianesi E. Carbohydrate intake and nonalcoholic fatty liver disease: fructose as a weapon of mass destruction. *Hepatobiliary Surg Nutr.* 2015; 4(2):109–116. doi:10.3978/j.issn.2304-3881.2014.11.05.

7. Sarkar D, Jung MK, Wang HJ. Alcohol and the Immune System. *Alcohol Res.* 2015; 37(2):153–155.

8. Alexopoulos N, Katritsis D, Raggi P. Visceral adipose tissue as a source of inflammation and promoter of atherosclerosis. *Atherosclerosis.* 2014; 233(1):104–112. doi:10.1016/j.atherosclerosis.2013.12.023.

9. Veldhuijzen van Zanten JJCS, Ring C, Carroll D, et al. Increased C reactive protein in response to acute stress in patients with rheumatoid arthritis. *Annals of the Rheumatic Diseases* 2005; 64:1299–1304.

10. Falconer CL, Cooper AR, Walhin JP, et al. Sedentary time and markers of inflammation in people with newly diagnosed type 2 diabetes. *Nutr Metab Cardiovasc Dis.* 2014; 24(9):956–962. doi:10.1016/j.numecd.2014.03.009.

11. Gao N, Xu W, Ji J, et al. Lung function and systemic inflammation associated with short-term air pollution exposure in chronic obstructive pulmonary disease patients in Beijing, China. *Environ Health* 19, 12 (2020). https://doi.org/10.1186/s12940-020-0568-1.

12. Rizzetto L, Fava F, Tuohy KM, Selmi C. Connecting the immune system, systemic chronic inflammation and the gut microbiome: The role of sex. *J Autoimmun*. 2018; 92:12–34. doi:10.1016/j.jaut.2018.05.008.

13. Roivainen M, Viik-Kajander M, Palosuo T, et al. Infections, inflammation, and the risk of coronary heart disease. *Circulation*. 2000; 101(3):252–257. doi:10.1161/01.cir.101.3.252.

14. Pothineni NVK, Subramany S, Kuriakose K, Shirazi LF, Romeo F, Shah PK, Mehta JL. Infections, atherosclerosis, and coronary heart disease, *European Heart Journal*, 2017; 38(43) :3195–3201. https://doi.org/10.1093/eurheartj/ehx362.

15. Rose NR. Infection, mimics, and autoimmune disease. *J Clin Invest*. 2001; 107(8):943–944. doi:10.1172/JCI12673.

16. Cunningham MW. Pathogenesis of Group A Streptococcal Infections. *Clinical Microbiology Reviews* Jul 2000, 13 (3) 470–511. doi: 10.1128/CMR.13.3.470.

17. James JA, Robertson JM. Lupus and Epstein-Barr. *Curr Opin Rheumatol*. 2012; 24(4):383–388. doi:10.1097/BOR.0b013e3283535801.

18. Singh SK, Girschick HJ. Lyme borreliosis: from infection to autoimmunity. *Clin Microbiol Infect*. 2004; 10(7):598–614. doi:10.1111/j.1469-0691.2004.00895.x.

19. Kalish RA, Leong JM, Steere AC. Association of treatment-resistant chronic Lyme arthritis with HLA-DR4 and antibody reactivity to OspA and OspB of Borrelia burgdorferi. *Infect Immun*. 1993; 61(7):2774-2779. doi:10.1128/IAI.61.7.2774-2779.1993.

20. Liu Y, Sawalha AH, Lu Q. COVID-19 and autoimmune diseases. *Curr Opin Rheumatol*. 2021; 33(2):155–162. doi:10.1097/BOR.0000000000000776.

21. Rehman S, Majeed T, Ansari MA, Al-Suhaimi EA. Syndrome resembling Kawasaki disease in COVID-19 asymptomatic children. *J Infect Public Health*. 2020; 13(12):1830–1832. doi:10.1016/j.jiph.2020.08.003.

22. Saad MA, Alfishawy M, Nassar M, Mohamed M, Esene IN, and Elbendary A, COVID-19 and Autoimmune Diseases: A Systematic Review of Reported Cases, *Current Rheumatology Reviews* (2021) 17:193. https://doi.org/10.2174/1573397116666201029155856.

23. Wang EY, Mao T, Klein J, et al. Diverse Functional Autoantibodies in Patients with COVID-19. Preprint. *medRxiv*. 2020; 2020.12.10.20247205. Published 2020 Dec 12. doi:10.1101/2020.12.10.20247205.

24. Rubin R. As Their Numbers Grow, COVID-19 "Long Haulers" Stump Experts. *JAMA*. 2020; 324(14):1381–1383. doi:10.1001/jama.2020.17709.

25. Mizushima N, Levine B, Cuervo AM, Klionsky DJ. Autophagy fights disease through cellular self-digestion. *Nature*. 2008; 451(7182):1069–1075. doi:10.1038/nature06639.

26. Levine B, Deretic V. Unveiling the roles of autophagy in innate and adaptive immunity. *Nat Rev Immunol*. 2007; 7(10):767–777. doi:10.1038/nri2161.

27. Funderburk SF, Marcellino BK, Yue Z. Cell "self-eating" (autophagy) mechanism in Alzheimer's disease. *Mt Sinai J Med*. 2010; 77(1):59–68. doi:10.1002/msj.20161.

28. Lünemann, J, Münz, C. Autophagy in CD4$^+$ T-cell immunity and tolerance. *Cell Death Differ* 16, 79–86 (2009). https://doi.org/10.1038/cdd.2008.113.

29. Yun CW, Lee SH. The Roles of Autophagy in Cancer. *Int J Mol Sci*. 2018; 19(11):3466. Published 2018 Nov 5. doi:10.3390/ijms19113466.

30. Nakamura S, Yoshimori T. Autophagy and Longevity. *Mol Cells*. 2018; 41(1):65–72. doi:10.14348/molcells.2018.2333.

31. Martinez-Lopez N, Tarabra E, Toledo M, et al. System-wide Benefits of Intermeal Fasting by Autophagy. *Cell Metab*. 2017; 26(6):856-871.e5. doi:10.1016/j.cmet.2017.09.020.

32. Choi IY, Lee C, Longo VD. Nutrition and fasting mimicking diets in the prevention and treatment of autoimmune diseases and immunosenescence. *Mol Cell Endocrinol*. 2017; 455:4–12. doi:10.1016/j.mce.2017.01.042.

Chapter 4: The Four Immunotypes Quiz

1. Rashid T, Ebringer A, Autoimmunity in Rheumatic Diseases Is Induced by Microbial Infections via Crossreactivity or Molecular Mimicry. *Autoimmune Diseases*. 2012, article ID 539282, 2012. https://doi.org/10.1155/2012/539282.

2. Park H, Li Z, Yang XO, et al. A distinct lineage of CD4 T cells regulates tissue inflammation by producing interleukin 17. *Nat Immunol*. 2005; 6(11): 1133–1141. doi:10.1038/ni1261.

3. Weaver CT, Harrington LE, Mangan PR, Gavrieli M, Murphy KM. Th17: an effector CD4 T cell lineage with regulatory T cell ties. *Immunity*. 2006 Jun; 24(6):677–88. doi: 10.1016/j.immuni.2006.06.002. PMID: 16782025.

4. Tesmer LA, Lundy SK, Sarkar S, Fox DA. Th17 cells in human disease. *Immunol Rev*. 2008; 223:87–113. doi:10.1111/j.1600-065X.2008.00628.x.

5. Yasuda K, Takeuchi Y, Hirota K. The pathogenicity of Th17 cells in autoimmune diseases. *Semin Immunopathol*. 2019 May; 41(3):283–297. doi: 10.1007

/s00281-019-00733-8. Epub 2019 Mar 19. Erratum in: *Semin Immunopathol.* 2019 Apr 29. PMID: 30891627.

6. Vignali DA, Collison LW, Workman CJ. How regulatory T cells work. *Nat Rev Immunol.* 2008; 8(7):523–532. doi:10.1038/nri2343.

Chapter 5: Sleep: Power Down Your Body, Power Up Your Immune System

1. Vitaterna MH, Takahashi JS, Turek FW. Overview of circadian rhythms. *Alcohol Res Health.* 2001; 25(2):85–93.

2. Comas M, Gordon CJ, Oliver BG, et al. A circadian based inflammatory response—implications for respiratory disease and treatment. *Sleep Science Practice* 1, 18 (2017). https://doi.org/10.1186/s41606-017-0019-2.

3. Carrillo-Vico A, Lardone PJ, Alvarez-Sánchez N, Rodríguez-Rodríguez A, Guerrero JM. Melatonin: buffering the immune system. *Int J Mol Sci.* 2013; 14(4):8638–8683. Published 2013 Apr 22. doi:10.3390/ijms14048638.

4. Provencio I, Jiang G, De Grip WJ, Hayes WP, Rollag MD. Melanopsin: An opsin in melanophores, brain, and eye. *Proc Natl Acad Sci USA.* 1998; 95(1):340–345. doi:10.1073/pnas.95.1.340.

5. Wahl S, Engelhardt M, Schaupp P, Lappe C, Ivanov IV. The inner clock -Blue light sets the human rhythm. *J Biophotonics.* 2019; 12(12):e201900102. doi:10.1002/jbio.201900102.

6. Gradisar M, Wolfson AR, Harvey AG, Hale L, Rosenberg R, Czeisler CA. The sleep and technology use of Americans: findings from the National Sleep Foundation's 2011 Sleep in America poll. *J Clin Sleep Med.* 2013; 9(12):1291–1299. Published 2013 Dec 15. doi:10.5664/jcsm.3272.

7. Chang AM, Aeschbach D, Duffy JF, Czeisler CA. Evening use of light -emitting eReaders negatively affects sleep, circadian timing, and next -morning alertness. *Proc Natl Acad Sci USA.* 2015; 112(4):1232–1237. doi:10.1073/pnas.1418490112.

8. Dimitrov S, Benedict C, Heutling D, Westermann J, Born J, Lange T. Cortisol and epinephrine control opposing circadian rhythms in T cell subsets. *Blood.* 2009;113(21):5134–5143. doi:10.1182/blood-2008-11-190769.

9. Besedovsky L, Lange T, Born J. Sleep and immune function. *Pflugers Arch.* 2012; 463(1):121–137. doi:10.1007/s00424-011-1044-0.

10. Mullington J, Korth C, Hermann DM, et al. Dose-dependent effects of endotoxin on human sleep. *Am J Physiol Regul Integr Comp Physiol.* 2000; 278(4):R947–R955. doi:10.1152/ajpregu.2000.278.4.R947.

11. Imeri L, Opp MR. How (and why) the immune system makes us sleep. *Nat Rev Neurosci.* 2009; 10(3):199–210. doi:10.1038/nrn2576.

12. Kluger MJ, Kozak W, Conn CA, Leon LR, Soszynski D. The adaptive value of fever. *Infect Dis Clin North Am.* 1996; 10(1):1–20. doi:10.1016/s0891 -5520(05)70282-8.

13. Reiter RJ, Mayo JC, Tan DX, Sainz RM, Alatorre-Jimenez M, Qin L. Melatonin as an antioxidant: under promises but over delivers. *J Pineal Res.* 2016; 61(3):253–278. doi:10.1111/jpi.12360.

14. Knutson KL, Spiegel K, Penev P, Van Cauter E. The metabolic consequences of sleep deprivation. *Sleep Med Rev.* 2007;11(3):163–178. doi:10.1016 /j.smrv.2007.01.002.

15. Spiegel K, Leproult R, Van Cauter E. Impact of sleep debt on metabolic and endocrine function. *Lancet.* 1999; 354(9188):1435–1439. doi:10.1016/S0140 -6736(99)01376-8.

16. Knutson KL. Impact of sleep and sleep loss on glucose homeostasis and appetite regulation. *Sleep Med Clin.* 2007; 2(2):187–197. doi:10.1016/j.jsmc.2007.03.004.

17. Dias JP, Joseph JJ, Kluwe B, et al. The longitudinal association of changes in diurnal cortisol features with fasting glucose: MESA. *Psychoneuroendocrinology.* 2020; 119:104698. doi:10.1016/j.psyneuen.2020.104698.

18. Sanyaolu A, Okorie C, Marinkovic A, et al. Comorbidity and its Impact on Patients with COVID-19 [published online ahead of print, 2020 Jun 25]. *SN Compr Clin Med.* 2020; 1–8. doi:10.1007/s42399-020-00363-4.

19. Chiappetta, S, Sharma, AM, Bottino, V, et al. COVID-19 and the role of chronic inflammation in patients with obesity. *Int J Obes* 44, 1790–1792 (2020). https://doi.org/10.1038/s41366-020-0597-4.

20. Lange T, Perras B, Fehm HL, Born J. Sleep enhances the human antibody response to hepatitis A vaccination. *Psychosom Med.* 2003; 65(5):831–835. doi:10.1097/01.psy.0000091382.61178.f1.

21. Taylor DJ, Kelly K, Kohut ML, Song KS. Is Insomnia a Risk Factor for Decreased Influenza Vaccine Response?. *Behav Sleep Med.* 2017; 15(4):270– 287. doi:10.1080/15402002.2015.1126596.

22. Cohen S, Doyle WJ, Alper CM, Janicki-Deverts D, Turner RB. Sleep habits and susceptibility to the common cold. *Arch Intern Med.* 2009; 169(1):62–67. doi:10.1001/archinternmed.2008.505.

23. Collins KP, Geller DA, Antoni M, et al. Sleep duration is associated with survival in advanced cancer patients. *Sleep Med.* 2017; 32:208–212. doi:10 .1016/j.sleep.2016.06.041.

24. Irwin M, McClintick J, Costlow C, Fortner M, White J, Gillin JC. Partial night sleep deprivation reduces natural killer and cellular immune responses in humans. *FASEB J.* 1996; 10(5):643–653. doi:10.1096/fasebj.10.5.8621064.

25. Hirshkowitz M, Whiton K, Albert SM, et al. National Sleep Foundation's sleep time duration recommendations: methodology and results summary. *Sleep Health.* 2015; 1(1):40–43. doi:10.1016/j.sleh.2014.12.010.

26. Haghayegh S, Khoshnevis S, Smolensky MH, Diller KR, Castriotta RJ. Before-bedtime passive body heating by warm shower or bath to improve sleep: A systematic review and meta-analysis. *Sleep Med Rev.* 2019; 46:124–135. doi:10.1016/j.smrv.2019.04.008.

27. Lillehei AS, Halcon LL. A systematic review of the effect of inhaled essential oils on sleep. *J Altern Complement Med.* 2014; 20(6):441–451. doi:10.1089/acm.2013.0311.

28. McDonnell B, Newcomb P. Trial of Essential Oils to Improve Sleep for Patients in Cardiac Rehabilitation. *J Altern Complement Med.* 2019; 25(12):1193–1199. doi:10.1089/acm.2019.0222.

29. Taibi DM, Vitiello MV. A pilot study of gentle yoga for sleep disturbance in women with osteoarthritis. *Sleep Med.* 2011; 12(5):512–517. doi:10.1016/j.sleep.2010.09.016.

30. Srivastava JK, Shankar E, Gupta S. Chamomile: A herbal medicine of the past with bright future. *Mol Med Rep.* 2010; 3(6):895–901. doi:10.3892/mmr.2010.377.

31. Ngan A, Conduit R. A double-blind, placebo-controlled investigation of the effects of Passiflora incarnata (passionflower) herbal tea on subjective sleep quality. *Phytother Res.* 2011; 25(8):1153–1159. doi:10.1002/ptr.3400.

32. Shechter A, Kim EW, St-Onge MP, Westwood AJ. Blocking nocturnal blue light for insomnia: A randomized controlled trial. *J Psychiatr Res.* 2018; 96:196–202. doi:10.1016/j.jpsychires.2017.10.015.

Chapter 6: Optimize Your Stress—the Good and the Bad

1. Goldstein DS, McEwen B. Allostasis, homeostats, and the nature of stress. *Stress.* 2002; 5(1):55–58. doi:10.1080/102538902900012345.

2. Moreno-Smith M, Lutgendorf SK, Sood AK. Impact of stress on cancer metastasis. *Future Oncol.* 2010; 6(12):1863–1881. doi:10.2217/fon.10.142.

3. Dimsdale JE. Psychological stress and cardiovascular disease. *J Am Coll Cardiol.* 2008; 51(13):1237–1246. doi:10.1016/j.jacc.2007.12.024.

4. Hammen C. Stress and depression. *Annu Rev Clin Psychol.* 2005; 1:293–319. doi:10.1146/annurev.clinpsy.1.102803.143938.

5. Song H, Fang F, Tomasson G, et al. Association of Stress-Related Disorders with Subsequent Autoimmune Disease. *JAMA.* 2018; 319(23):2388–2400. doi:10.1001/jama.2018.7028.

6. Dhabhar FS. Effects of stress on immune function: the good, the bad, and the beautiful. *Immunol Res.* 2014; 58(2–3):193–210. doi:10.1007/s12026-014-8517-0.

7. Hassett AL, Clauw DJ. The role of stress in rheumatic diseases. *Arthritis Res Ther.* 2010; 12(3):123. doi:10.1186/ar3024.

8. Mawdsley JE, Rampton DS. Psychological stress in IBD: new insights into pathogenic and therapeutic implications. *Gut.* 2005; 54(10):1481–1491. doi:10.1136/gut.2005.064261.

9. Suárez AL, Feramisco JD, Koo J, Steinhoff M. Psychoneuroimmunology of psychological stress and atopic dermatitis: pathophysiologic and therapeutic updates. *Acta Derm Venereol.* 2012; 92(1):7–15. doi:10.2340/00015555-1188.

10. Chen E, Miller GE. Stress and inflammation in exacerbations of asthma. *Brain Behav Immun.* 2007; 21(8):993–999. doi:10.1016/j.bbi.2007.03.009.

11. Dhabhar FS, Malarkey WB, Neri E, McEwen BS. Stress-induced redistribution of immune cells—from barracks to boulevards to battlefields: a tale of three hormones—Curt Richter Award winner. *Psychoneuroendocrinology.* 2012; 37(9):1345–1368. doi:10.1016/j.psyneuen.2012.05.008.

12. Nieman DC, Wentz LM. The compelling link between physical activity and the body's defense system. *J Sport Health Sci.* 2019; 8(3):201–217. doi:10.1016/j.jshs.2018.09.009.

13. Evans ES, Hackney AC, McMurray RG, et al. Impact of Acute Intermittent Exercise on Natural Killer Cells in Breast Cancer Survivors. *Integr Cancer Ther.* 2015; 14(5):436–445. doi:10.1177/1534735415580681.

14. Ford, ES. Does Exercise Reduce Inflammation? Physical Activity and C-Reactive Protein Among U.S. Adults, *Epidemiology:* 2002; 13(5): 561–568.

15. Edwards KM, Burns VE, Reynolds T, Carroll D, Drayson M, Ring C. Acute stress exposure prior to influenza vaccination enhances antibody response in women. *Brain Behav Immun.* 2006; 20(2):159–168. doi:10.1016/j.bbi.2005.07.001.

16. Campbell JP, Turner JE. Debunking the Myth of Exercise-Induced Immune Suppression: Redefining the Impact of Exercise on Immunological Health

Across the Lifespan. *Front Immunol*. 2018; 9:648. Published 2018 Apr 16. doi:10.3389/fimmu.2018.00648.

17. Friedenreich CM. Physical activity and cancer prevention: from observational to intervention research. *Cancer Epidemiol Biomarkers Prev*. 2001; 10(4): 287–301.

18. Beavers KM, Brinkley TE, Nicklas BJ. Effect of exercise training on chronic inflammation. *Clin Chim Acta*. 2010; 411(11–12):785-793. doi:10.1016/j.cca.2010.02.069.

19. da Silveira MP, da Silva Fagundes KK, Bizuti MR, Starck É, Rossi RC, de Resende E Silva DT. Physical exercise as a tool to help the immune system against COVID-19: an integrative review of the current literature. *Clin Exp Med*. 2021; 21(1):15–28. doi:10.1007/s10238-020-00650-3.

20. Morey JN, Boggero IA, Scott AB, Segerstrom SC. Current Directions in Stress and Human Immune Function. *Curr Opin Psychol*. 2015; 5:13–17. doi:10.1016/j.copsyc.2015.03.007.

21. Chandola T, Brunner E, Marmot M. Chronic stress at work and the metabolic syndrome: prospective study. *BMJ*. 2006; 332(7540):521–525. doi:10.1136/bmj.38693.435301.80.

22. Kivimäki M, Kawachi I. Work Stress as a Risk Factor for Cardiovascular Disease. *Curr Cardiol Rep*. 2015; 17(9):630. doi:10.1007/s11886-015-0630-8.

23. Saul AN, Oberyszyn TM, Daugherty C, et al. Chronic stress and susceptibility to skin cancer. *J Natl Cancer Inst*. 2005; 97(23):1760–1767. doi:10.1093/jnci/dji401.

24. Moreno-Smith M, Lutgendorf SK, Sood AK. Impact of stress on cancer metastasis. *Future Oncol*. 2010; 6(12):1863–1881. doi:10.2217/fon.10.142.

25. Bookwalter DB, Roenfeldt KA, LeardMann CA, et al. Posttraumatic stress disorder and risk of selected autoimmune diseases among US military personnel. *BMC Psychiatry* 20, 23 (2020). https://doi.org/10.1186/s12888-020-2432-9.

26. Dube SR, Fairweather D, Pearson WS, Felitti VJ, Anda RF, Croft JB. Cumulative childhood stress and autoimmune diseases in adults. *Psychosom Med*. 2009; 71(2):243–250. doi:10.1097/PSY.0b013e3181907888.

27. Zannas AS, West AE. Epigenetics and the regulation of stress vulnerability and resilience. *Neuroscience*. 2014; 264:157–170. doi:10.1016/j.neuroscience.2013.12.003.

28. Black DS, Slavich GM. Mindfulness meditation and the immune system: a systematic review of randomized controlled trials. *Ann N Y Acad Sci.* 2016; 1373(1):13–24. doi:10.1111/nyas.12998.

29. Haluza D, Schönbauer R, Cervinka R. Green perspectives for public health: a narrative review on the physiological effects of experiencing outdoor nature. *Int J Environ Res Public Health.* 2014; 11(5):5445–5461. Published 2014 May 19. doi:10.3390/ijerph110505445.

30. Peluso MA, Guerra de Andrade LH. Physical activity and mental health: the association between exercise and mood. *Clinics (Sao Paulo).* 2005; 60(1):61–70. doi:10.1590/s1807-59322005000100012.

31. Anderson T, Lane AR, Hackney AC. Cortisol and testosterone dynamics following exhaustive endurance exercise. *Eur J Appl Physiol.* 2016; 116(8):1503–1509. doi:10.1007/s00421-016-3406-y.

32. Takayama F, Aoyagi A, Takahashi K, Nabekura Y. Relationship between oxygen cost and C-reactive protein response to marathon running in college recreational runners. *Open Access J Sports Med.* 2018; 9:261–268. Published 2018 Nov 27. doi:10.2147/OAJSM.S183274.

33. Anderson T, Lane AR, Hackney AC. Cortisol and testosterone dynamics following exhaustive endurance exercise. *Eur J Appl Physiol.* 2016 Aug; 116(8):1503–9. doi: 10.1007/s00421-016-3406-y. Epub 2016 Jun 4. PMID: 27262888.

34. Kreher JB, Schwartz JB. Overtraining syndrome: a practical guide. *Sports Health.* 2012; 4(2):128–138. doi:10.1177/1941738111434406.

35. Panossian AG, Efferth T, Shikov AN, et al. Evolution of the adaptogenic concept from traditional use to medical systems: Pharmacology of stress- and aging-related diseases. *Med Res Rev.* 2021; 41(1):630–703. doi:10.1002/med.21743.

36. Li Y, Pham V, Bui M, et al. *Rhodiola rosea L.:* an herb with anti-stress, anti-aging, and immunostimulating properties for cancer chemoprevention. *Curr Pharmacol Rep.* 2017; 3(6):384–395. doi:10.1007/s40495-017-0106-1.

37. Cicero AF, Derosa G, Brillante R, Bernardi R, Nascetti S, Gaddi A. Effects of Siberian ginseng (Eleutherococcus senticosus maxim) on elderly quality of life: a randomized clinical trial. *Arch Gerontol Geriatr Suppl.* 2004; (9):69–73. doi:10.1016/j.archger.2004.04.012.

38. Panossian A, Wikman G. Effects of Adaptogens on the Central Nervous System and the Molecular Mechanisms Associated with Their Stress-Protective Activity. *Pharmaceuticals (Basel).* 2010; 3(1):188–224. Published 2010 Jan 19. doi:10.3390/ph3010188.

39. Chandrasekhar K, Kapoor J, Anishetty S. A prospective, randomized double-blind, placebo-controlled study of safety and efficacy of a high-concentration full-spectrum extract of ashwagandha root in reducing stress and anxiety in adults. *Indian J Psychol Med*. 2012; 34(3):255–262. doi:10.4103 /0253-7176.106022.

40. Baek JH, Heo JY, Fava M, et al. Effect of Korean Red Ginseng in individuals exposed to high stress levels: a 6-week, double-blind, randomized, placebo-controlled trial. *J Ginseng Res*. 2019; 43(3):402–407. doi:10.1016 /j.jgr.2018.03.001.

41. Scholey A, Gibbs A, Neale C, et al. Anti-stress effects of lemon balm-containing foods. *Nutrients*. 2014 ;6(11):4805–4821. Published 2014 Oct 30. doi:10.3390/nu6114805.

42. Talbott SM, Talbott JA, Pugh M. Effect of Magnolia officinalis and Phellodendron amurense (Relora®) on cortisol and psychological mood state in moderately stressed subjects. *J Int Soc Sports Nutr*. 2013; 10(1):37. Published 2013 Aug 7. doi:10.1186/1550-2783-10-37.

Chapter 7: Tend to Your GALT—the Home of Your Immune System

1. Nagler-Anderson C. Man the barrier! Strategic defences in the intestinal mucosa. *Nat Rev Immunol*. 2001; 1(1):59–67. doi:10.1038/35095573.

2. Vighi G, Marcucci F, Sensi L, Di Cara G, Frati F. Allergy and the gastrointestinal system. *Clin Exp Immunol*. 2008; 153 Suppl 1(Suppl 1):3–6. doi:10 .1111/j.1365-2249.2008.03713.x.

3. Sender R, Fuchs S, Milo R. Revised Estimates for the Number of Human and Bacteria Cells in the Body. *PLoS Biol*. 2016; 14(8):e1002533. Published 2016 Aug 19. doi:10.1371/journal.pbio.1002533.

4. Lyon L. "All disease begins in the gut": was Hippocrates right? *Brain*. March 2018; 141(3): e20. https://doi.org/10.1093/brain/awy017.

5. Lloyd-Price J, Abu-Ali G, Huttenhower C. The healthy human microbiome. *Genome Med*. 2016; 8(1):51. Published 2016 Apr 27. doi:10.1186/s13073 -016-0307-y.

6. O'Hara AM, Shanahan F. The gut flora as a forgotten organ. *EMBO Rep*. 2006; 7(7):688–693. doi:10.1038/sj.embor.7400731.

7. Tamburini S, Shen N, Wu H., et al. The microbiome in early life: implications for health outcomes. *Nat Med* 22, 713–722 (2016). https://doi.org /10.1038/nm.4142.

8. Belkaid Y, Hand TW. Role of the microbiota in immunity and inflammation. *Cell.* 2014; 157(1):121–141. doi:10.1016/j.cell.2014.03.011.

9. Troy EB, Kasper DL. Beneficial effects of Bacteroides fragilis polysaccharides on the immune system. *Front Biosci (Landmark Ed).* 2010; 15:25–34. Published 2010 Jan 1. doi:10.2741/3603.

10. Ege MJ. The Hygiene Hypothesis in the Age of the Microbiome. *Ann Am Thorac Soc.* 2017; 14(Supplement_5):S348-S353. doi:10.1513/AnnalsATS .201702-139AW.

11. Lazar V, Ditu LM, Pircalabioru GG, et al. Aspects of Gut Microbiota and Immune System Interactions in Infectious Diseases, Immunopathology, and Cancer. *Front Immunol.* 2018; 9:1830. Published 2018 Aug 15. doi:10.3389 /fimmu.2018.01830.

12. Kamada N, Chen GY, Inohara N, Núñez G. Control of pathogens and pathobionts by the gut microbiota. *Nat Immunol.* 2013; 14(7):685–690. doi:10.1038/ni.2608.

13. Baldini F, Hertel J, Sandt E, et al. Parkinson's disease-associated alterations of the gut microbiome predict disease-relevant changes in metabolic functions. *BMC Biol.* 2020; 18(1):62. Published 2020 Jun 9. doi:10.1186/s12915 -020-00775-7.

14. Kowalski K, Mulak A. Brain-Gut-Microbiota Axis in Alzheimer's Disease. *J Neurogastroenterol Motil.* 2019; 25(1):48–60. doi:10.5056/jnm18087.

15. Knight-Sepulveda K, Kais S, Santaolalla R, Abreu MT. Diet and Inflammatory Bowel Disease. *Gastroenterol Hepatol (N Y).* 2015; 11(8):511–520.

16. Devkota S, Wang Y, Musch MW, et al. Dietary-fat-induced taurocholic acid promotes pathobiont expansion and colitis in Il10-/- mice. *Nature.* 2012; 487(7405):104–108. doi:10.1038/nature11225.

17. Strober W. Adherent-invasive E. coli in Crohn disease: bacterial "agent provocateur." *J Clin Invest.* 2011; 121(3):841–844. doi:10.1172/JCI46333.

18. Yue B, Luo X, Yu Z, Mani S, Wang Z, Dou W. Inflammatory Bowel Disease: A Potential Result from the Collusion between Gut Microbiota and Mucosal Immune System. *Microorganisms.* 2019; 7(10):440. Published 2019 Oct 11. doi:10.3390/microorganisms7100440.

19. Horta-Baas G, Romero-Figueroa MDS, Montiel-Jarquín AJ, Pizano -Zárate ML, García-Mena J, Ramírez-Durán N. Intestinal Dysbiosis and Rheumatoid Arthritis: A Link between Gut Microbiota and the Pathogenesis of Rheumatoid Arthritis. *J Immunol Res.* 2017; 2017:4835189. doi:10.1155 /2017/4835189.

20. Gill T, Asquith M, Rosenbaum JT, Colbert RA. The intestinal microbiome in spondyloarthritis. *Curr Opin Rheumatol.* 2015; 27(4):319–325. doi:10.1097/BOR.0000000000000187.

21. Codoñer FM, Ramírez-Bosca A, Climent E, et al. Gut microbial composition in patients with psoriasis. *Sci Rep.* 2018; 8(1):3812. Published 2018 Feb 28. doi:10.1038/s41598-018-22125-y.

22. Jie Z, Xia H, Zhong SL, et al. The gut microbiome in atherosclerotic cardiovascular disease. *Nat Commun.* 2017; 8(1):845. Published 2017 Oct 10. doi:10.1038/s41467-017-00900-1.

23. Gurung M, Li Z, You H, et al. Role of gut microbiota in type 2 diabetes pathophysiology. *EBioMedicine.* 2020; 51:102590. doi:10.1016/j.ebiom.2019.11.051.

24. Jin M, Qian Z, Yin J, Xu W, Zhou X. The role of intestinal microbiota in cardiovascular disease. *J Cell Mol Med.* 2019; 23(4):2343–2350. doi:10.1111/jcmm.14195.

25. Fasano A. Zonulin and its regulation of intestinal barrier function: the biological door to inflammation, autoimmunity, and cancer. *Physiol Rev.* 2011; 91(1):151–175. doi:10.1152/physrev.00003.2008.

26. Fasano A. Intestinal permeability and its regulation by zonulin: diagnostic and therapeutic implications. *Clin Gastroenterol Hepatol.* 2012; 10(10):1096–1100. doi:10.1016/j.cgh.2012.08.012.

27. Barbaro MR, Cremon C, Morselli-Labate AM, et al. Serum zonulin and its diagnostic performance in non-coeliac gluten sensitivity. *Gut* 2020; 69:1966–1974.

28. Talpaert MJ, Gopal Rao G, Cooper BS, Wade P. Impact of guidelines and enhanced antibiotic stewardship on reducing broad-spectrum antibiotic usage and its effect on incidence of Clostridium difficile infection. *J Antimicrob Chemother.* 2011; 66(9):2168–2174. doi:10.1093/jac/dkr253.

29. Ktsoyan Z, Budaghyan L, Agababova M, et al. Potential Involvement of *Salmonella* Infection in Autoimmunity. *Pathogens.* 2019; 8(3):96. Published 2019 Jul 3. doi:10.3390/pathogens8030096.

30. Quagliani D, Felt-Gunderson P. Closing America's fiber intake gap: communication strategies from a food and fiber summit. *Am J Lifestyle Med.* 2016; 11(1):80–85. Published 2016 Jul 7. doi:10.1177/1559827615588079.

31. Zimmer J, Lange B, Frick JS, et al. A vegan or vegetarian diet substantially alters the human colonic faecal microbiota. *Eur J Clin Nutr.* 2012; 66(1):53–60. doi:10.1038/ejcn.2011.141.

32. Wu X, Wu Y, He L, Wu L, Wang X, Liu Z. Effects of the intestinal microbial metabolite butyrate on the development of colorectal cancer. *J Cancer.* 2018; 9(14):2510–2517. Published 2018 Jun 15. doi:10.7150/jca.25324.

33. Mesnage R, Teixeira M, Mandrioli D, et al. Use of shotgun metagenomics and metabolomics to evaluate the impact of glyphosate or Roundup MON 52276 on the gut microbiota and serum metabolome of Sprague-Dawley rats. *Environ Health Perspect.* 2021; 129(1):17005. doi:10.1289/EHP6990.

34. Kogevinas M. Probable carcinogenicity of glyphosate *BMJ* 2019; 365:l1613 doi:10.1136/bmj.l1613.

35. Hemarajata P, Versalovic J. Effects of probiotics on gut microbiota: mechanisms of intestinal immunomodulation and neuromodulation. *Therap Adv Gastroenterol.* 2013; 6(1):39–51. doi:10.1177/1756283X12459294.

Chapter 8: Toxins — The Ultimate Immune System Distracters

1. Thompson PA, Khatami M, Baglole CJ, et al. Environmental immune disruptors, inflammation and cancer risk. *Carcinogenesis.* 2015; 36 Suppl 1(Suppl 1):S232–S253. doi:10.1093/carcin/bgv038.

2. Dietert RR, Etzel RA, Chen D, et al. Workshop to identify critical windows of exposure for children's health: immune and respiratory systems work group summary. *Environ Health Perspect.* 2000; 108 Suppl 3(Suppl 3):483–490. doi:10.1289/ehp.00108s3483.

3. Winans B, Humble MC, Lawrence BP. Environmental toxicants and the developing immune system: a missing link in the global battle against infectious disease? *Reprod Toxicol.* 2011; 31(3):327–336. doi:10.1016/j.reprotox .2010.09.004.

4. Braun KM, Cornish T, Valm A, Cundiff J, Pauly JL, Fan S. Immunotoxicology of cigarette smoke condensates: suppression of macrophage responsiveness to interferon gamma. *Toxicol Appl Pharmacol.* 1998 Apr; 149(2):136v43. doi: 10.1006/taap.1997.8346. PMID: 9571981.

5. Stevens EA, Mezrich JD, Bradfield CA. The aryl hydrocarbon receptor: a perspective on potential roles in the immune system. *Immunology.* 2009; 127(3):299–311. doi:10.1111/j.1365-2567.2009.03054.x.

6. Robinson L, Miller R. The impact of bisphenol A and phthalates on allergy, asthma, and immune function: a review of latest findings. *Curr Environ Health Rep.* 2015; 2(4):379–387. doi:10.1007/s40572-015-0066-8.

7. Le Magueresse-Battistoni B, Vidal H, Naville D. Environmental pollutants

and metabolic disorders: the multi-exposure scenario of life. *Front Endocrinol (Lausanne)*. 2018; 9:582. Published 2018 Oct 2. doi:10.3389/fendo.2018.00582.

8. Sobel ES, Gianini J, Butfiloski EJ, Croker BP, Schiffenbauer J, Roberts SM. Acceleration of autoimmunity by organochlorine pesticides in (NZB x NZW)F1 mice. *Environ Health Perspect*. 2005 Mar; 113(3):323–8. doi: 10.1289/ehp.7347. PMID: 15743722; PMCID: PMC1253759.

9. Cooper GS, Wither J, Bernatsky S, et al. Occupational and environmental exposures and risk of systemic lupus erythematosus: silica, sunlight, solvents. *Rheumatology (Oxford)*. 2010; 49(11):2172–2180. doi:10.1093/rheumatology/keq214.

10. Blake BE, Fenton SE. Early life exposure to per- and polyfluoroalkyl substances (PFAS) and latent health outcomes: A review including the placenta as a target tissue and possible driver of peri- and postnatal effects. *Toxicology*. 2020; 443:152565. doi:10.1016/j.tox.2020.152565.

11. Mon Monograph: Perfluorooctanoic Acid or Perfluorooctane Sulfonate; Sept. 2016. *National Toxicology Program US Department of Health and Human Services*.

12. Domingo JL, Nadal M. Human exposure to per- and polyfluoroalkyl substances (PFAS) through drinking water: A review of the recent scientific literature. *Environ Res*. 2019 Oct; 177:108648. doi: 10.1016/j.envres.2019.108648. Epub 2019 Aug 12. PMID: 31421451.

13. Vojdani A, Pollard KM, Campbell AW. Environmental triggers and autoimmunity. *Autoimmune Dis*. 2014; 2014:798029. doi:10.1155/2014/798029.

14. Quirós-Alcalá L, Hansel NN, McCormack MC, Matsui EC. Paraben exposures and asthma-related outcomes among children from the US general population. *J Allergy Clin Immunol*. 2019; 143(3):948–956.e4. doi:10.1016/j.jaci.2018.08.021.

15. Larsson M, Hägerhed-Engman L, Kolarik B, James P, Lundin F, Janson S, Sundell J, Bornehag CG. PVC—as flooring material—and its association with incident asthma in a Swedish child cohort study. *Indoor Air*. 2010 Dec; 20(6):494–501. doi: 10.1111/j.1600-0668.2010.00671.x. PMID: 21070375.

16. Elter E, Wagner M, Buchenauer L, Bauer M, Polte T. Phthalate Exposure during the prenatal and lactational period increases the susceptibility to rheumatoid arthritis in mice. *Front Immunol*. 2020 Apr 3; 11:550. doi: 10.3389/fimmu.2020.00550. PMID: 32308655; PMCID: PMC7145968.

17. Darbre PD, Harvey PW. Parabens can enable hallmarks and characteristics of cancer in human breast epithelial cells: a review of the literature with reference to new exposure data and regulatory status. *J Appl Toxicol*. 2014 Sep; 34(9):925–38. doi: 10.1002/jat.3027. Epub 2014 Jul 22. PMID: 25047802.

18. Savage JH, Matsui EC, Wood RA, Keet CA. Urinary levels of triclosan and parabens are associated with aeroallergen and food sensitization. *J Allergy Clin Immunol.* 2012; 130(2):453–60.e7. doi:10.1016/j.jaci.2012.05.006.

19. Overexposed. Environmental Working Group. Accessed April 25, 2021. https://www.ewg.org/research/overexposed-organophosphate-insecticides -childrens-food.

20. Malagón-Rojas JN, Parra Barrera EL, Lagos L. From environment to clinic: the role of pesticides in antimicrobial resistance. *Rev Panam Salud Publica.* 2020; 44:e44. Published 2020 Sep 23. doi:10.26633/RPSP.2020.44.

21. Gangemi S, Gofita E, Costa C, et al. Occupational and environmental exposure to pesticides and cytokine pathways in chronic diseases (Review). *Int J Mol Med.* 2016; 38(4):1012–1020. doi:10.3892/ijmm.2016.2728.

22. Litteljohn D, Mangano E, Clarke M, Bobyn J, Moloney K, Hayley S. Inflammatory mechanisms of neurodegeneration in toxin-based models of Parkinson's disease. *Parkinsons Dis.* 2010; 2011:713517. Published 2010 Dec 30. doi:10.4061/2011/713517.

23. Lee GH, Choi KC. Adverse effects of pesticides on the functions of immune system. *Comp Biochem Physiol C Toxicol Pharmacol.* 2020 Sep; 235:108789. doi: 10.1016/j.cbpc.2020.108789. Epub 2020 May 3. PMID: 32376494.

24. Nayak AS, Lage CR, Kim CH. Effects of low concentrations of arsenic on the innate immune system of the zebrafish (Danio rerio). *Toxicol Sci.* 2007 Jul; 98(1):118–24. doi: 10.1093/toxsci/kfm072. Epub 2007 Mar 30. PMID: 17400579.

25. Skoczyńska A, Poreba R, Sieradzki A, Andrzejak R, Sieradzka U. Wpływ ołowiu i kadmu na funkcje układu immunologicznego [The impact of lead and cadmium on the immune system]. *Med Pr.* 2002; 53(3):259-64. Polish. PMID: 12369510.

26. Silva IA, Nyland JF, Gorman A, et al. Mercury exposure, malaria, and serum antinuclear/antinucleolar antibodies in Amazon populations in Brazil: a cross-sectional study. *Environ Health.* 2004; 3(1):11. Published 2004 Nov 2. doi:10.1186/1476-069X-3-11.

27. Silva IA, Nyland JF, Gorman A, et al. Mercury exposure, malaria, and serum antinuclear/antinucleolar antibodies in Amazon populations in Brazil: a cross-sectional study. *Environ Health.* 2004;3 (1):11. Published 2004 Nov 2. doi:10.1186/1476-069X-3-11.

28. Hodges RE, Minich DM. Modulation of Metabolic Detoxification Pathways Using Foods and Food-Derived Components: A Scientific Review

with Clinical Application. *J Nutr Metab.* 2015; 2015:760689. doi:10.1155 /2015/760689.

29. Eylar E, Rivera-Quinones C, Molina C, Báez I, Molina F, Mercado CM. *N*-Acetylcysteine enhances T cell functions and T cell growth in culture, *International Immunology,* 1983; 5(1): 97–101. https://doi.org/10.1093/intimm/5.1.97.

30. Polonikov A. Endogenous Deficiency of Glutathione as the Most Likely Cause of Serious Manifestations and Death in COVID-19 Patients. *ACS Infect Dis.* 2020; 6(7):1558–1562. doi:10.1021/acsinfecdis.0c00288.

31. Eliaz I, Weil E, Wilk B. Integrative medicine and the role of modified citrus pectin/alginates in heavy metal chelation and detoxification–five case reports. *Forschende Komplementarmedizin.* 2007; 14(6):358–364.

32. Uchikawa T, Kumamoto Y, Maruyama I, Kumamoto S, Ando Y, Yasutake A. The enhanced elimination of tissue methylmercury in Parachlorella beijerinckii-fed mice. *Journal of Toxicological Sciences.* 2011; 36(1):121–126.

33. Zellner T, Prasa D, Färber E, Hoffmann-Walbeck P, Genser D, Eyer F. The use of activated charcoal to treat intoxications. *Dtsch Arztebl Int.* 2019; 116(18):311–317. doi:10.3238/arztebl.2019.0311.

34. Kraljević Pavelić S, Simović Medica J, Gumbarević D, Filošević A, Pržulj N, Pavelić K. Critical review on zeolite clinoptilolite safety and medical applications *in vivo. Front Pharmacol.* 2018; 9:1350. Published 2018 Nov 27. doi:10.3389/fphar.2018.01350.

Chapter 9: Nutrition—Feeding Your Immune System

1. Obukhov AG, Stevens BR, Prasad R, Li Calzi S, Boulton ME, Raizada MK, Oudit GY, Grant MB. SARS-CoV-2 infections and ACE2: Clinical outcomes linked with increased morbidity and mortality in individuals with diabetes. *Diabetes.* 2020 Sep; 69(9):1875–1886. doi: 10.2337/dbi20 -0019. Epub 2020 Jul 15. PMID: 32669391; PMCID: PMC7458035.

2. Alcock J, Maley CC, Aktipis CA. Is eating behavior manipulated by the gastrointestinal microbiota? Evolutionary pressures and potential mechanisms. *Bioessays.* 2014; 36(10):940–949. doi:10.1002/bies.201400071.

3. How much sugar is too much? www.heart.org. Accessed April 25, 2021. https://www.heart.org/en/healthy-living/healthy-eating/eat-smart/sugar /how-much-sugar-is-too-much.

4. Jung ES, Park JI, Park H, Holzapfel W, Hwang JS, Lee CH. Seven-day green tea supplementation revamps gut microbiome and caecum/skin

metabolome in mice from stress. *Sci Rep.* 2019 Dec 5; 9(1):18418. doi: 10.1038/s41598-019-54808-5. PMID: 31804534; PMCID: PMC6895175.

5. Bungau S, Abdel-Daim MM, Tit DM, et al. Health benefits of polyphenols and carotenoids in age-related eye diseases. *Oxid Med Cell Longev.* 2019; 2019:9783429. Published 2019 Feb 12. doi:10.1155/2019/9783429.

6. Wu D. Green tea EGCG, T-cell function, and T-cell-mediated autoimmune encephalomyelitis. *J Investig Med.* 2016 Dec; 64(8):1213–1219. doi: 10.1136/jim-2016-000158. Epub 2016 Aug 16. PMID: 27531904.

7. Chaplin A, Carpéné C, Mercader J. Resveratrol, metabolic syndrome, and gut microbiota. *Nutrients.* 2018; 10(11):1651. Published 2018 Nov 3. doi:10 .3390/nu10111651.

8. Lin R, Piao M, Song Y. Dietary quercetin increases colonic microbial diversity and attenuates colitis severity in *Citrobacter rodentium*-infected mice. *Front Microbiol.* 2019; 10:1092. Published 2019 May 16. doi:10.3389 /fmicb.2019.01092.

9. Jafarinia M, Sadat Hosseini M, Kasiri N, et al. Quercetin with the potential effect on allergic diseases. *Allergy Asthma Clin Immunol.* 2020; 16:36. Published 2020 May 14. doi:10.1186/s13223-020-00434-0.

10. Chambial S, Dwivedi S, Shukla KK, John PJ, Sharma P. Vitamin C in disease prevention and cure: an overview. *Indian J Clin Biochem.* 2013; 28(4):314 -328. doi:10.1007/s12291-013-0375-3.

11. Hemilä H, de Man AME. Vitamin C and COVID-19. *Front Med (Lausanne).* 2021; 7:559811. Published 2021 Jan 18. doi:10.3389/fmed.2020 .559811.

12. de Melo AF, Homem-de-Mello M. High-dose intravenous vitamin C may help in cytokine storm in severe SARS-CoV-2 infection. *Critical Care.* 2020; 24(1). doi:10.1186/s13054-020-03228-3.

13. Ran L, Zhao W, Wang J, et al. Extra dose of vitamin C based on a daily supplementation shortens the common cold: A meta-analysis of 9 randomized controlled trials. *Biomed Res Int.* 2018; 2018:1837634. Published 2018 Jul 5. doi:10.1155/2018/1837634.

14. Office of Dietary Supplements, National Institutes of Health Dietary Supplement Fact Sheet: Vitamin E. From: www.ods.od.nih.gov/factsheets /vitamine.asp Accessed: Aug 2010.

15. Kalayci O, Besler T, Kilinç K, Sekerel BE, Saraçlar Y. Serum levels of antioxidant vitamins (alpha tocopherol, beta carotene, and ascorbic acid) in

children with bronchial asthma. *Turk J Pediatr.* 2000 Jan–Mar; 42(1):17-21. PMID: 10731863.

16. Meydani SN, Leka LS, Fine BC, et al. Vitamin E and respiratory tract infections in elderly nursing home residents: a randomized controlled trial [published correction appears in *JAMA.* 2004 Sep 15; 292(11):1305] [published correction appears in *JAMA.* 2007 May 2; 297(17):1882]. *JAMA.* 2004; 292(7):828-836. doi:10.1001/jama.292.7.828.

17. Bungau S, Abdel-Daim MM, Tit DM, et al. Health benefits of polyphenols and carotenoids in age-related eye diseases. *Oxid Med Cell Longev.* 2019; 2019:9783429. Published 2019 Feb 12. doi:10.1155/2019/9783429.

18. Huang Z, Liu Y, Qi G, Brand D, Zheng SG. Role of vitamin A in the immune system. *J Clin Med.* 2018; 7(9):258. Published 2018 Sep 6. doi:10.3390/jcm7090258.

19. Al Senaidy AM. Serum vitamin A and beta-carotene levels in children with asthma. *J Asthma.* 2009 Sep; 46(7):699–702. doi: 10.1080/02770900903056195. PMID: 19728208.

20. Schambach F, Schupp M, Lazar MA, Reiner SL. Activation of retinoic acid receptor-alpha favours regulatory T cell induction at the expense of IL-17-secreting T helper cell differentiation. *Eur J Immunol.* 2007 Sep; 37(9):2396–9. doi: 10.1002/eji.200737621. PMID: 17694576.

21. Czarnewski P, Das S, Parigi SM, Villablanca EJ. Retinoic acid and its role in modulating intestinal innate immunity. *Nutrients.* 2017 Jan 13; 9(1):68. doi: 10.3390/nu9010068. PMID: 28098786; PMCID: PMC5295112.

22. Leung WC, Hessel S, Méplan C, Flint J, Oberhauser V, Tourniaire F, Hesketh JE, von Lintig J, Lietz G. Two common single nucleotide polymorphisms in the gene encoding beta-carotene 15,15'-monoxygenase alter beta-carotene metabolism in female volunteers. *FASEB J.* 2009 Apr; 23(4):1041–53. doi: 10.1096/fj.08-121962. Epub 2008 Dec 22. PMID: 19103647.

23. Omeed Sizar, Swapnil Khare, Amandeep Goyal, Pankaj Bansal, Givler A. Vitamin D deficiency. Published January 3, 2021. https://www.ncbi.nlm.nih.gov/books/NBK532266/.

24. Garland CF, Kim JJ, Mohr SB, et al. Meta-analysis of all-cause mortality according to serum 25-hydroxyvitamin D. *Am J Public Health.* 2014; 104(8): e43-e50. doi:10.2105/AJPH.2014.302034.

25. Prietl B, Pilz S, Wolf M, Tomaschitz A, Obermayer-Pietsch B, Graninger W, Pieber TR. Vitamin D supplementation and regulatory T cells in

apparently healthy subjects: vitamin D treatment for autoimmune diseases? *Isr Med Assoc J.* 2010 Mar; 12(3):136-9. PMID: 20684175.

26. Cantorna MT, Snyder L, Lin YD, Yang L. Vitamin D and 1,25(OH)2D regulation of T cells. *Nutrients.* 2015; 7(4):3011–3021. Published 2015 Apr 22. doi:10.3390/nu7043011.

27. Pierrot-Deseilligny C, Souberbielle JC. Contribution of vitamin D insufficiency to the pathogenesis of multiple sclerosis. *Ther Adv Neurol Disord.* 2013; 6(2):81–116. doi:10.1177/1756285612473513.

28. Bhutta ZA. Vitamin D reduces respiratory tract infections frequency. *J Pediatrics.* 2017; 186:209–212. doi:10.1016/j.jpeds.2017.04.021.

29. Combs GF Jr. Status of selenium in prostate cancer prevention. *Br J Cancer.* 2004; 91(2):195–199. doi:10.1038/sj.bjc.6601974.

30. Huang Z, Rose AH, Hoffmann PR. The role of selenium in inflammation and immunity: from molecular mechanisms to therapeutic opportunities. *Antioxid Redox Signal.* 2012; 16(7):705–743. doi:10.1089/ars.2011.4145.

31. Wood SM, Beckham C, Yosioka A, Darban H, Watson RR. Beta-Carotene and selenium supplementation enhances immune response in aged humans. *Integr Med.* 2000 Mar 21; 2(2):85-92. doi: 10.1016/s1096-2190(00)00009-3. PMID: 10882881.

32. World Health Organization. The World Health report 2002. *Midwifery.* (2003) 19:72–3. 10.1054/midw.2002.0343.

33. Wessels I, Maywald M, Rink L. Zinc as a gatekeeper of immune function. *Nutrients.* 2017; 9(12):1286. Published 2017 Nov 25. doi:10.3390/nu 9121286.

34. Rao G, Rowland K. PURLs: Zinc for the common cold—not if, but when. *J Fam Pract.* 2011; 60(11):669–671.

35. Novak M, Vetvicka V. Beta-glucans, history, and the present: immunomodulatory aspects and mechanisms of action. *J Immunotoxicol.* 2008 Jan; 5(1):47–57. doi: 10.1080/15476910802019045. PMID: 18382858.

36. Shin MS, Park HJ, Maeda T, Nishioka H, Fujii H, Kang I. The effects of AHCC®, a standardized extract of cultured *Lentinura edodes* mycelia, on natural killer and t cells in health and disease: Reviews on human and animal studies. *J Immunol Res.* 2019; 2019:3758576. Published 2019 Dec 20. doi:10.1155/2019/3758576.

37. Murphy EJ, Masterson C, Rezoagli E, et al. β-Glucan extracts from the same edible shiitake mushroom Lentinus edodes produce differential in-vitro immunomodulatory and pulmonary cytoprotective effects—Implications for coro-

navirus disease (COVID-19) immunotherapies. *Sci Total Environ.* 2020; 732:139330. doi:10.1016/j.scitotenv.2020.139330.

38. Saleh MH, Rashedi I, Keating A. Immunomodulatory properties of *Coriolus versicolor*: The Role of polysaccharopeptide. *Front Immunol.* 2017 Sep 6; 8:1087. doi: 10.3389/fimmu.2017.01087. PMID: 28932226; PMCID: PMC 5592279.

39. Guggenheim AG, Wright KM, Zwickey HL. Immune modulation from five major mushrooms: Application to integrative oncology. *Integr Med (Encinitas).* 2014; 13(1):32–44.

40. Wachtel-Galor S, Yuen J, Buswell JA, et al. Ganoderma lucidum (Lingzhi or Reishi): A medicinal mushroom. In: Benzie IFF, Wachtel-Galor S, editors. *Herbal Medicine: Biomolecular and Clinical Aspects.* 2nd edition. Boca Raton (FL): CRC Press/Taylor & Francis; 2011. Chapter 9. Available from: https://www.ncbi.nlm.nih.gov/books/NBK92757/?report=classic.

41. Hewlings SJ, Kalman DS. Curcumin: A review of its effects on human health. *Foods.* 2017; 6(10):92. Published 2017 Oct 22. doi:10.3390/foods 6100092.

42. Burge K, Gunasekaran A, Eckert J, Chaaban H. Curcumin and intestinal inflammatory diseases: Molecular mechanisms of protection. *Int J Mol Sci.* 2019; 20(8):1912. Published 2019 Apr 18. doi:10.3390/ijms20081912.

43. Enyeart JA, Liu HL, Enyeart JJ. Curcumin inhibits ACTH- and angiotensin II-stimulated cortisol secretion and Ca(v)3.2 current. *J Nat Prod.* 2009; 72(8): 1533–1537. doi:10.1021/np900227x.

44. Shen L, Liu L, Ji HF. Regulative effects of curcumin spice administration on gut microbiota and its pharmacological implications. *Food Nutr. Res.* 2017; 61:1361780. doi: 10.1080/16546628.2017.1361780.

45. Brück J, Holstein J, Glocova I, et al. Nutritional control of IL-23/Th17 -mediated autoimmune disease through HO-1/STAT3 activation. *Sci Rep.* 2017 Mar 14; 7:44482. doi: 10.1038/srep44482. PMID: 28290522; PMCID: PMC5349589.

46. Shep D, Khanwelkar C, Gade P, et al. Safety and efficacy of curcumin versus diclofenac in knee osteoarthritis: a randomized open-label parallel-arm study. *Trials* 20, 214 (2019). https://doi.org/10.1186/s13063-019-3327-2.

47. Dai Q, Zhou D, Xu L, Song X. Curcumin alleviates rheumatoid arthritis -induced inflammation and synovial hyperplasia by targeting mTOR pathway in rats. *Drug Des Devel Ther.* 2018; 12:4095-4105. Published 2018 Dec 3. doi:10.2147/DDDT.S175763.

48. Nicoll R, Henein MY. Ginger (Zingiber officinale Roscoe): a hot remedy for cardiovascular disease? *Int J Cardiol.* 2009 Jan 24; 131(3):408–9. doi: 10.1016/j.ijcard.2007.07.107. Epub 2007 Nov 26. PMID: 18037515.

49. Mallikarjuna K, Sahitya Chetan P, Sathyavelu Reddy K, Rajendra W. Ethanol toxicity: rehabilitation of hepatic antioxidant defense system with dietary ginger. *Fitoterapia.* 2008 Apr; 79(3):174–8. doi: 10.1016/j.fitote.2007.11.007. Epub 2007 Nov 29. PMID: 18182172.

50. Ajith TA, Nivitha V, Usha S. Zingiber officinale Roscoe alone and in combination with alpha-tocopherol protect the kidney against cisplatin-induced acute renal failure. *Food Chem Toxicol.* 2007 Jun; 45(6):921–7. doi: 10.1016/j.fct.2006.11.014. Epub 2006 Nov 29. PMID: 17210214.

51. Karuppiah P, Rajaram S. Antibacterial effect of Allium sativum cloves and Zingiber officinale rhizomes against multiple-drug resistant clinical pathogens. *Asian Pac J Trop Biomed.* 2012; 2(8):597–601. doi:10.1016/S2221-1691(12)60104-X.

52. Mara Teles A, Araújo dos Santos B, Gomes Ferreira C, et al. Ginger (Zingiber officinale) antimicrobial potential: A review. *Ginger Cultivation and Its Antimicrobial and Pharmacological Potentials.* Published online February 19, 2020. Accessed April 25, 2021. http://dx.doi.org/10.5772/intechopen.89780.

53. Nikkhah Bodagh M, Maleki I, Hekmatdoost A. Ginger in gastrointestinal disorders: A systematic review of clinical trials. *Food Sci Nutr.* 2018; 7(1): 96–108. Published 2018 Nov 5. doi:10.1002/fsn3.807.

54. Vomund S, Schäfer A, Parnham MJ, Brüne B, von Knethen A. Nrf2, the master regulator of anti-oxidative responses. *Int J Mol Sci.* 2017; 18(12):2772. Published 2017 Dec 20. doi:10.3390/ijms18122772.

55. Fahey JW, Zhang Y, Talalay P. Broccoli sprouts: An exceptionally rich source of inducers of enzymes that protect against chemical carcinogens. *Proc Natl Acad Sci USA* Sep 1997, 94 (19) 10367–10372; DOI: 10.1073/pnas.94.19.10367.

56. López-Chillón MT, Carazo-Díaz C, Prieto-Merino D, Zafrilla P, Moreno DA, Villaño D. Effects of long-term consumption of broccoli sprouts on inflammatory markers in overweight subjects. *Clin Nutr.* 2019 Apr; 38(2):745–752. doi: 10.1016/j.clnu.2018.03.006. Epub 2018 Mar 13. PMID: 29573889.

57. Arreola R, Quintero-Fabián S, López-Roa RI, et al. Immunomodulation and anti-inflammatory effects of garlic compounds. *J Immunol Res.* 2015; 2015:401630. doi:10.1155/2015/401630.

58. Varshney R, Budoff MJ. Garlic and heart disease, *J Nutrition*. 2016; 146(2): 416S–421S.https://doi.org/10.3945/jn.114.202333.

59. Bayan L, Koulivand PH, Gorji A. Garlic: a review of potential therapeutic effects. *Avicenna J Phytomed*. 2014; 4(1):1–14.

Chapter 10: Rebalancing Your Immunotype

1. Guggenheim AG, Wright KM, Zwickey HL. Immune modulation from five major mushrooms: Application to integrative oncology. *Integr Med (Encinitas)*. 2014; 13(1):32–44.

2. Cardwell G, Bornman JF, James AP, Black LJ. A review of mushrooms as a potential source of dietary vitamin D. *Nutrients*. 2018;10(10):1498. Published 2018 Oct 13. doi:10.3390/nu10101498.

3. Falandysz J. Selenium in edible mushrooms. *J Environ Sci Health C Environ Carcinog Ecotoxicol Rev*. 2008 Jul–Sep; 26(3):256–99. doi: 10.1080/10590 500802350086. PMID: 18781538.

4. Salve J, Pate S, Debnath K, Langade D. Adaptogenic and anxiolytic effects of ashwagandha root extract in healthy adults: A double-blind, randomized, placebo-controlled clinical study. *Cureus*. 2019; 11(12):e6466. Published 2019 Dec 25. doi:10.7759/cureus.6466.

5. Grudzien M, Rapak A. Effect of natural compounds on NK cell activation. *J Immunol Res*. 2018 Dec 25; 2018:4868417. doi: 10.1155/2018/4868417. PMID: 30671486; PMCID: PMC6323526.

6. Khan S, Malik F, Suri KA, Singh J. Molecular insight into the immune up-regulatory properties of the leaf extract of Ashwagandha and identification of Th1 immunostimulatory chemical entity. *Vaccine*. 2009 Oct 9; 27(43):6080– 7. doi: 10.1016/j.vaccine.2009.07.011. Epub 2009 Jul 21. PMID: 19628058.

7. Saba E, Lee, Kim M, Kim SH, Hong SB, Rhee MH. A comparative study on immune-stimulatory and antioxidant activities of various types of ginseng extracts in murine and rodent models. *J Ginseng Res*. 2018; 42(4):577– 584. doi:10.1016/j.jgr.2018.07.004.

8. Ulfman LH, Leusen JHW, Savelkoul HFJ, Warner JO, van Neerven RJJ. Effects of bovine immunoglobulins on immune function, allergy, and infection. *Front Nutr*. 2018; 5:52. Published 2018 Jun 22. doi:10.3389/fnut .2018.00052.

9. Hałasa M, Maciejewska D, Baśkiewicz-Hałasa M, Machaliński B, Safranow K, Stachowska E. Oral supplementation with bovine colostrum decreases

intestinal permeability and stool concentrations of zonulin in athletes. *Nutrients.* 2017; 9(4):370. Published 2017 Apr 8. doi:10.3390/nu9040370.

10. Patıroğlu T, Kondolot M. The effect of bovine colostrum on viral upper respiratory tract infections in children with immunoglobulin A deficiency. *Clin Respir J.* 2013 Jan; 7(1):21–6. doi: 10.1111/j.1752-699X.2011.00268.x. Epub 2011 Sep 6. PMID: 21801330.

11. Velikova T, Tumangelova-Yuzeir K, Georgieva R, et al. Lactobacilli supplemented with larch arabinogalactan and colostrum stimulates an immune response towards peripheral NK activation and gut tolerance. *Nutrients.* 2020; 12(6):1706. Published 2020 Jun 7. doi:10.3390/nu12061706.

12. Riede L, Grube B, Gruenwald J. Larch arabinogalactan effects on reducing incidence of upper respiratory infections. *Curr Med Res Opin.* 2013; 29(3): 251–8. doi: 10.1185/03007995.2013.765837.

13. Barak V, Halperin T, Kalickman I. The effect of Sambucol, a black elderberry-based natural product, on the production of human cytokines: I. Inflammatory cytokines. *Eur Cytokine Netw.* 2001 Apr–Jun;12(2):290–6. PMID: 11399518.

14. Kunnumakkara AB, Bordoloi D, Padmavathi G, et al. Curcumin, the golden nutraceutical: multitargeting for multiple chronic diseases. *Br J Pharmacol.* 2017; 174(11):1325–1348. doi:10.1111/bph.13621.

15. Stohs SJ, Chen O, Ray SD, Ji J, Bucci LR, Preuss HG. Highly bioavailable forms of curcumin and promising avenues for curcumin-based research and application: A review. *Molecules.* 2020; 25(6):1397. Published 2020 Mar 19. doi:10.3390/molecules25061397.

16. Ramírez-Garza SL, Laveriano-Santos EP, Marhuenda-Muñoz M, et al. Health effects of resveratrol: Results from human intervention trials. *Nutrients.* 2018; 10(12):1892. Published 2018 Dec 3. doi:10.3390/nu10121892.

17. Movahed A, Nabipour I, Lieben Louis X, et al. Antihyperglycemic effects of short term resveratrol supplementation in type 2 diabetic patients. *Evid Based Complement Alternat Med.* 2013; 2013:851267. doi:10.1155/2013/851267.

18. Rahman MH, Akter R, Bhattacharya T, et al. Resveratrol and neuroprotection: Impact and its therapeutic potential in Alzheimer's disease. *Front Pharmacol.* 2020; 11:619024. Published 2020 Dec 30. doi:10.3389/fphar.2020.619024.

19. Timmers S, Konings E, Bilet L, et al. Calorie restriction–like effects of 30 days of resveratrol supplementation on energy metabolism and metabolic profile in obese humans. *Cell Metab.* 2011; 14(5):612–622. doi:10.1016/j.cmet.2011.10.002.

20. Li Z, Geng YN, Jiang JD, Kong WJ. Antioxidant and anti-inflammatory activities of berberine in the treatment of diabetes mellitus. *Evid Based Complement Alternat Med.* 2014; 2014:289264. doi:10.1155/2014/289264.

21. Yin J, Xing H, Ye J. Efficacy of berberine in patients with type 2 diabetes mellitus. *Metabolism.* 2008; 57(5):712–717. doi:10.1016/j.metabol.2008.01.013.

22. Deo SS, Mistry KJ, Kakade AM, Niphadkar PV. Role played by Th2 type cytokines in IgE mediated allergy and asthma. *Lung India.* 2010; 27(2):66–71. doi:10.4103/0970-2113.63609.

23. Mlcek J, Jurikova T, Skrovankova S, Sochor J. Quercetin and its anti-allergic immune response. *Molecules.* 2016; 21(5):623. Published 2016 May 12. doi:10.3390/molecules21050623.

24. Wang W, Jing W, Liu Q. *Astragalus* oral solution ameliorates allergic asthma in children by regulating relative contents of CD4[+]CD25[high]CD127[low] Treg cells. *Front Pediatr.* 2018; 6:255. Published 2018 Sep 20. doi:10.3389/fped.2018.00255.

25. Chen SM, Tsai YS, Lee SW, Liu YH, Liao SK, Chang WW, Tsai PJ. Astragalus membranaceus modulates Th1/2 immune balance and activates PPARγ in a murine asthma model. *Biochem Cell Biol.* 2014 Oct; 92(5):397–405. doi:10.1139/bcb-2014-0008. Epub 2014 Sep 2. PMID: 25264079.

26. Takano H, Osakabe N, Sanbongi C, et al. Extract of Perilla frutescens enriched for rosmarinic acid, a polyphenolic phytochemical, inhibits seasonal allergic rhinoconjunctivitis in humans. *Experimental Biology and Medicine.* 2004; 229(3):247–254.

27. Bakhshaee M, Mohammad Pour AH, Esmaeili M, et al. Efficacy of supportive therapy of allergic rhinitis by stinging nettle *(Urtica dioica)* root extract: A randomized, double-blind, placebo-controlled, clinical trial. *Iran J Pharm Res.* 2017; 16(Suppl):112–118.

28. Chandrasekaran A, Molparia B, Akhtar E, et al. The autoimmune protocol diet modifies intestinal RNA expression in inflammatory bowel disease. *Crohns Colitis 360.* 2019; 1(3):otz016. doi:10.1093/crocol/otz016.

29. Bakdash G, Vogelpoel LT, van Capel TM, Kapsenberg ML, de Jong EC. Retinoic acid primes human dendritic cells to induce gut-homing, IL-10-producing regulatory T cells. *Mucosal Immunol.* 2015 Mar; 8(2):265–78. doi:10.1038/mi.2014.64. Epub 2014 Jul 16. PMID: 25027601.

30. Elias KM, Laurence A, Davidson TS, et al. Retinoic acid inhibits Th17 polarization and enhances FoxP3 expression through a Stat-3/Stat-5 independent signaling pathway. *Blood.* 2008; 111(3):1013v1020. doi:10.1182/blood-2007-06-096438.

31. Bastos MS, Rolland Souza AS, Costa Caminha MF, et al. Vitamin A and pregnancy: A narrative review. *Nutrients*. 2019; 11(3):681. Published 2019 Mar 22. doi:10.3390/nu11030681.

32. Krakauer T, Li BQ, Young HA. The flavonoid baicalin inhibits superantigen-induced inflammatory cytokines and chemokines. *FEBS Lett*. 2001 Jun 29; 500(1–2):52–5. doi: 10.1016/s0014-5793(01)02584-4. PMID: 11434925.

33. Yang J, Yang X, Yang J, Li M. Baicalin ameliorates lupus autoimmunity by inhibiting differentiation of Tfh cells and inducing expansion of Tfr cells. *Cell Death Dis*. 2019; 10(2):140. Published 2019 Feb 13. doi:10.1038/s41419-019-1315-9.

34. Liang S, Deng X, Lei L, et al. The comparative study of the therapeutic effects and mechanism of baicalin, baicalein, and their combination on ulcerative colitis rat. *Front Pharmacol*. 2019; 10:1466. Published 2019 Dec 13. doi:10.3389/fphar.2019.01466.

35. Wu J, Li H, Li M. Effects of baicalin cream in two mouse models: 2,4-dinitrofluorobenzene-induced contact hypersensitivity and mouse tail test for psoriasis. *Int J Clin Exp Med*. 2015 Feb 15; 8(2):2128–37. PMID: 25932143; PMCID: PMC4402790.

36. Kurniawan H, Franchina DG, Guerra L, et al. Glutathione restricts serine metabolism to preserve regulatory T cell function. *Cell Metab*. 2020 May 5; 31(5):920-936.e7. doi: 10.1016/j.cmet.2020.03.004. Epub 2020 Mar 25. PMID: 32213345; PMCID: PMC7265172.

37. Kadry MO. Liposomal glutathione as a promising candidate for immunological rheumatoid arthritis therapy. *Heliyon*. 2019; 5(7):e02162. Published 2019 Jul 27. doi:10.1016/j.heliyon.2019.e02162.

38. Cascão R, Fonseca JE, Moita LF. Celastrol: A spectrum of treatment opportunities in chronic diseases. *Front Med* (Lausanne). 2017 Jun 15; 4:69. doi: 10.3389/fmed.2017.00069. PMID: 28664158; PMCID: PMC5471334.

39. Ibid.

40. Wang HL, Jiang Q, Feng XH, et al. Tripterygium wilfordii Hook F versus conventional synthetic disease-modifying anti-rheumatic drugs as monotherapy for rheumatoid arthritis: a systematic review and network meta-analysis. *BMC Complement Altern Med*. 2016; 16:215. Published 2016 Jul 13. doi:10.1186/s12906-016-1194-x.

41. Baek SY, Lee J, Lee DG, et al. Ursolic acid ameliorates autoimmune arthritis via suppression of Th17 and B cell differentiation. *Acta Pharmacol Sin*. 2014; 35(9):1177–1187. doi:10.1038/aps.2014.58.

Chapter 11: The Immune Restoration Plan at a Glance

1. Strindhall J, Nilsson BO, Löfgren S, et al. No Immune Risk Profile among individuals who reach 100 years of age: findings from the Swedish NONA immune longitudinal study. *Exp Gerontol.* 2007; 42(8):753–761. doi:10.1016/j.exger.2007.05.001.

2. Sabetta JR, DePetrillo P, Cipriani RJ, Smardin J, Burns LA, Landry ML. Serum 25-hydroxyvitamin D and the incidence of acute viral respiratory tract infections in healthy adults. *PLoS One.* 2010; 5(6):e11088. Published 2010 Jun 14. doi:10.1371/journal.pone.0011088.

3. Grant WB, Lahore H, McDonnell SL, et al. Evidence that Vitamin D supplementation could reduce risk of influenza and COVID-19 infections and deaths. *Nutrients.* 2020; 12(4):988. Published 2020 Apr 2. doi:10.3390/nu12040988.

Index

About the Author

Dr. Heather Moday is a board–certified allergist and immunologist, as well as an integrative and functional medicine physician. After years of working as an allergist and immunologist in private practice, she completed a fellowship in integrative medicine at the Arizona Center for Integrative Medicine in Tucson and became certified by the Institute for Functional Medicine. She is part of the mindbodygreen "Collective"—the wellness website's curated group of the top fifty experts in the wellness space. Through her practice, the Moday Center, she works to empower people to reclaim their health through comprehensive lifestyle programs, which focus on reversing chronic disease, as well as creating optimum wellness. She lives in Virginia with her partner and their cats, Flannel and Raphael, and dog, Remi. She can be followed on Instagram @theimmunityMD and Facebook @modaycenter215.